RELIGION SOCIAL CHANGE AND FERTILITY BEHAVIOUR

RELIGION SOCIAL CHANGE AND FERTILITY BEHAVIOUR

A Study of Kerala

R. JAYASREE

With an Introduction by
Prof. K. Mahadevan

CONCEPT PUBLISHING COMPANY, NEW DELHI-110059

The responsibility for the facts stated, conclusions reached and opinions expressed in this work is entirely that of the author and not of the Indian Council of Social Science Research which has financed the publication of this work.

ISBN 81-7022-252-4

First Published 1989

R. **Jayasree** (*b*. 1957-)

Published by
Ashok Kumar Mittal
Concept Publishing Company
A/15-16, Commercial Block, Mohan Garden
NEW DELHI-110059 (India)

Lasertypeset by
Microtech Advance Printing Systems (P) Ltd.
H-13, Bali Nagar, NEW DELHI-110015

Printed in India at
A.P. Offset Punchsheel Garden,
Naveen Shahdara Delhi-32

DEDICATED

TO

Prof. John C. Caldwell

Director, Department of Demography
Australian National University
Canberra

CONTENTS

PREFACE

Though the genesis of fertility studies in Kerala goes back to as early as the 1960s, a gap of research still exists on several aspects of fertility to explain the complete determinants of the exceptionally low fertility paradoxically seen in this economically poor state in the Indian Union. No doubt, several of the earlier studies broadly explained a few important determinants of fertility behaviour (Kurup and George, 1965; Nayar, 1974 & 1983; Zachariah, 1983; Namboodiri, 1986; Mahadevan, 1986 & 1987). They include widespread education, late marriage, occupational mobility, migration, status of women, modernization and family planning. But these factors had been studied on a random basis in the population, without stratifying the society on the basis of religion, caste, or class. Despite the socialist and communist influence in this state during the last four decades, Kerala society continues to be stratified on the basis of religion, though class distinction has narrowed down very much after independence. Of course, religious differences have not much affected the harmonious way of life of the people. In Kerala, so far, no major research has focussed on the differential influence of the determinants of fertility among the different religious groups. The aim of the present research is to study the determinants of fertility behaviour viz., Age at marriage, contraception, Breastfeeding, Birth interval, socio-economic factors and value of children that influence fertility behaviour, besides social change that happened among the population of the Travancore Region of Kerala in India. These differences were studied across the three major religious groups viz., the Hindus, Muslims and Christians inorder to assess the differential influence of various determinants of fertility among them. Therefore, it is ideal to consider these well known major determinants of fertility along with the new factors across these groups. However, in order to focus the study on a deeper basis only a few crucial variables have been considered for the present.

The Travancore region is the Southern most erstwhile kingdom of the present Kerala State. This region is purposely selected for the presence of all the religious groups and also because it manifests significant differential fertility. Kerala came into being with the amalgamation of three former princely states, viz., Travancore, Cochin and Malabar. The demographic Scenario of Kerala has become world famous, because in spite of the limited economic development, the crude birth rate has fallen to 24 per thousand live births by 1984. According to the 1981 census crude birth rate was 26.4 per thousand live births. This level of low birth rate is equivalent to the rates prevailing in the several developed countries. Certain studies have explained the major contributory factors of the rapid decline of fertility in this state since independence (1947). A recent study commissioned by the Central Health and Family Welfare Ministry confirmed that differential fertility exists across different religious groups in Kerala (Mahadevan 1987), which provides the justification for undertaking this present investigation. This study proved that despite high level of modernization and social change, cultural diversity and demographic differences are very conspicuous among the different religious groups. Hence, it is a priority and innovative area, to explore the unexplained determinants of cross-cultural fertility differences in Kerala.

The conceptual basis of the present study is focussed on several theoretical contributions on intermediate variables made by Davis and Blake (1956), proximate determinants of fertility by Bongaarts (1978), modified conceptual model of Freedman by Ruth Simmons et al., (1983), and the one very recently developed by Mahadevan and Sumangala (1986). The main dependent variable is live births, and the several independent variables have been considered on the basis of the models discussed above. For the selection of sample a multistage random sampling procedure was followed. As a first step of sampling Trivandrum District was selected purposely because of its representative character with most of the other districts in Travancore Region. As a second stage of selection of sample, three community development blocks from the Trivandrum District viz., Athiyannoor, Chirayinkil and Vellanadu were selected, again at random. Out of these three Community Development Blocks, villages were listed out serially and selected three villages each till the sufficient number of sample was obtained. Thus 1000 eligible couples constitute the respondents and among the couples wives were only

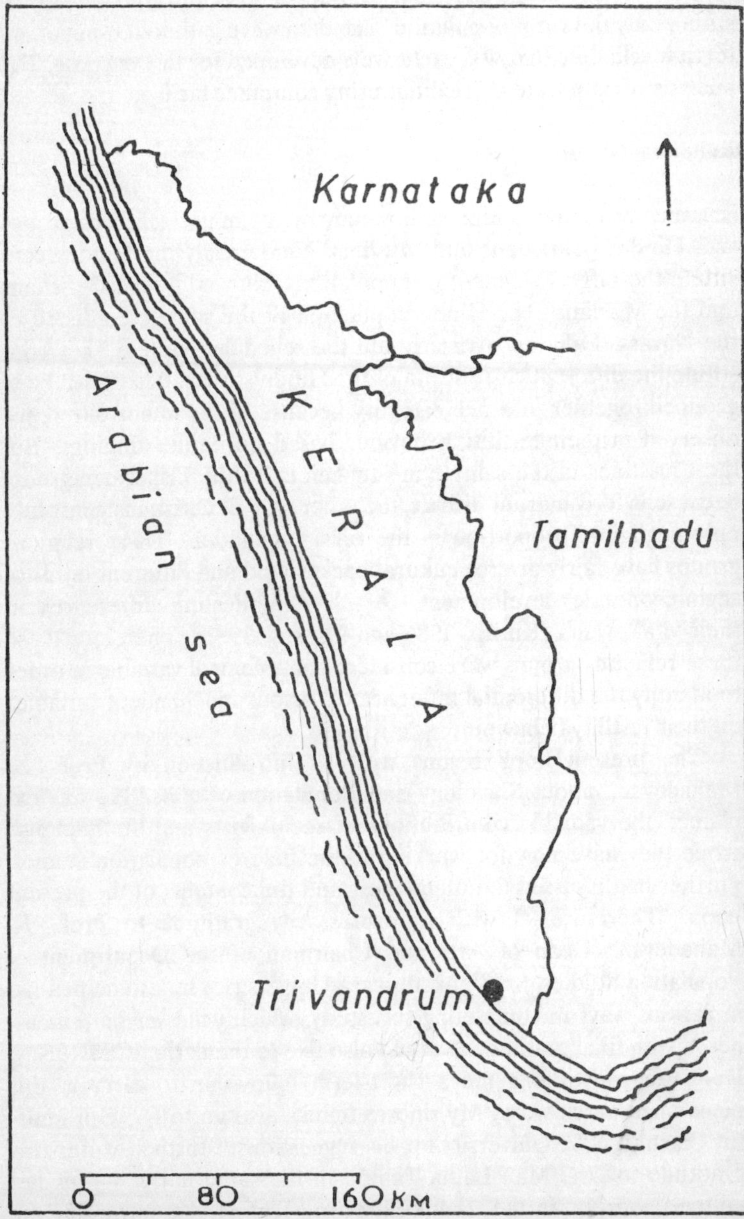
Karnataka
KERALA
Tamilnadu
Arabian sea
Trivandrum
0
80
160 KM

interviewed for data collection. The universe of the study also constitute only the rural population. The data were gathered using an interview schedule that was exclusively developed for this purpose. The analysis of data were carried out using computer facility.

Religious Groups

Travancore region is inhabited mainly by the major religious groups viz., Hindus, Christians and Muslims. Numerically the Hindus constitute the largest segment of population, followed by the Christians and the Muslims. The Hindu population of the sample consisted of the Nayars, Ezhavas, Artisans and the scheduled castes. They constitute the different caste strata of the Hindu society. They have been grouped together into one category because of the minor difference observed in their fertility behaviour based on earlier findings. But the Christians of the sample mostly belong to the Fishermen group, because in Trivandrum district, the other type of christians constitute only negligible proportion in the rural population. These religious groups have fairly diverse cultural background and different levels of socio-economic development, besides manifesting differences in their vital events (Kurup, 1986 and Census, 1981). Therefore these three religious groups were considered as a control variable in order to identify the differential influence of various independent variables on their fertility behaviour.

The present book begins with an introduction by Prof. K. Mahadevan, about Sociology and Population Studies. He has explained the valuable contributions of sociologists and the immense scope they have now for working in the field of population studies. Further he discussed the uniqueness and the contents of the present book. Therefore, I wish to express my gratitude to Prof. K. Mahadevan, Dean of Arts and Chairman of the Department of Population Studies, Sri Venkateswara University. He also helped me in various ways in completing this study, which will ever be remembered with filial gratitude. I would also like to thank the ICSSR, New Delhi for sanctioning me a short-term fellowship to carryout this piece of research work. My sincere thanks also go to Dr. Gurumurthy, Faculty, S.V. University for his suggestions. I further express my gratitude to Dr. (Ms.) Latha Tampi, of the same university for her editorial work. I further thank Director, T.I.F.R. for providing me computer facility for tabulating the data. My thanks are also due to

Sri Venkateswara University, Tirupati and the Department of Population Studies of the same University for permitting me to publish this book out of the data that I used for my Doctoral Programme.

Coimbatore
New Year Day, 1989

R. JAYASREE

INTRODUCTION

Sociology and Population Studies

K. Mahadevan

Population studies continues to depend increasingly on Sociology and other sister Social Sciences for its theoretical basis, methodological applications, adoption of relevant concepts for the study of population phenomena, knowledge for the successful promotion of population control programme and for the improvement of the quality of life of the population in general. The ideas drawn from social sciences make population studies as an applied as well as a dynamic subject for specialised purpose of studying population problem, and for promoting effective and suitable interventions to control the rapid growth of population. Although population studies has become an independent profession in several countries, its dependence on sociology will continue for ever. The nature of their dependence however, varies from country to country according to the background of the people who gave leadership to this profession. For instance, population studies continues to remain a sub-discipline of sociology either in the departments of Sociology or independently as in the case of most American Universities, since the leadership for this profession in U.S.A. was given largely by sociologists like Kingsley Davis, Ronald Freedman, Bernard Berelson, Mayon Stycos, Ruben Hill, Krishnan Namboodiri, Everett M. Rogers and several others. Besides sociologists, economists, anthropologists, psychologists, geographers, statisticians, mathematicians and public health personnels also gave a lead to this profession in certain universities in America, Europe and in developing countries.

According to Wilbert E. Moore (1959: 832), population studies in U.S.A. owe a great deal to sociology for its development and growth. He wrote: "At least in American college organization, demography is allocated to sociology more frequently than to other disciplines. The majority of courses are offered in sociology departments, and sociology is consequently the formal field in which at least a plurality of practising demographers have received advanced degrees .... Whether the American student of sociology specializes in demography or not, he is at least likely to get some elementary introduction to the study of population in several sociology courses. Most of the standard "introductory" or "principal" texts in sociology have larger or smaller sections explicitly devoted to population size and composition, fertility, mortality and migration. The level of theoretical and methodological sophistication in the treatment of demographic subjects is of course highly variable among the widely-used texts. The primary point of present interest is not the adequacy of their introduction to technical field but rather the fact that the attempt is made to treat demography as a subfield of sociology."

But the situation in India is different because the initial leadership was given in this course by scholars from the field of statistics, medicine, economics and to a negligible extent by sociology. The contribution of sociologists and other social scientists to the population studies in India gained momentum only from the 1970's. If the present trend continues, social scientists will increasingly play a dominant role in the years to come for promoting population studies in this country. A retrospective review of the best contributions made so far in major areas of population studies viz., (i) Fertility, (ii) Family planning, (iii) Mortality, (iv) Migration and Urbanization; and (v) Population Education-cum-Cummunication have been considered here. The contributions of social scientists from India and elsewhere to population studies dominates over the other similar efforts made by scholars in medical and mathematical sciences. Of course, the mathematical demographers have made a substantial contribution to the field of Evaluation of Family Planning and building of models on Fertility and Mortality, but not in the other core areas of different dimensions of population studies mentioned above. On the other hand, the Medical Science continues to contribute additional knowledge largely in the field of contraceptive technology, service and follow-up of contraceptives, follow-up studies in the form of evaluation and specialised studies on causes of death in the field of mortality. Except these efforts, most of the other major and valuable contributions made in the field of studies on Fertility, Mortality, Family Planning, Migration and Urbanization and Population Education and Communication have been made by sociologists and other sister social scientists. In the following pages an attempt has been made to focus the salient and specialised contributions made by social scientists in general and by sociologists in particular for the promotion of population studies.

Sociology and General Population Theory

A number of general theories on population have been postulated by sociologists as well as by economists. A retrospective glance at the theories formulated by sociologists will be very appropriate here to focus attention on the theoretical contributions of sociologists to Population studies. A succinct discussion on this aspect is given lucidly in a U.N. document on "The Determinants and Consequences of Population Trends" (1973). It stated "A number of late 19th and early 20th century sociological theories considered the relationship between population growth and concentration and the evolution and progress of society. According to some of these, human communities, while they grow in volume and density, experience progress in the form of the development of the division of labour, the extension of personal contacts and coordination of individual activities; the stimulation of initiative and technical innovations and the creation of other conditions which together make up social progress and the development of civilization" (Mougeolle, 1883; Giddings, 1896).

"Coste was among those who held that actual social evolution, as distinct from what he termed ideological phenomena, is the result of the growth of population and increase in its density (Coste, 1900). Durkheim held that the transformation of segmentary societies into population growth in organically well-knit communities is brought about by and the subsequent development of division of the labour. The growth and condensation of societies require a more far-reaching division of labour, which can be attained more rapidly the faster the number of individuals increases (Durkheim 1893). More recently, Dupreel and his school stressed the importance of population growth for technical and social progress and for the consequent raising of the cultural and material levels of living. According to this thesis, population growth produces effects such as the augmentation of social mobility; increases the frequency of personal contacts and in consequence, in social and intellectual stimuli; changes in values including greater emphasis on the future; a more optimistic and enterprising climate of expectation, and intensified technological progress and innovation.... A number of writers have speculated about the interrelations between the decline in fertility in the economically more developed countries and social conditions. Noting that this phenomenon spread simultaneously with changes in social environments, they enumerated such factors, as the diversification of man's activities, his increasing individuality, his growing concern with well-being and the more widespread employment of women. Factors associated with the urbanization process and the growing spirit of rationalization were discussed as relevant to the shaping of attitudes in favour of reducing the size of families (Nitti, 1984; Spengler, 1921; Mombert, 1912).

A theory on this basis was developed by Dumont, who formulated the principle of "Social Capillarity". He, like number of other writers before him, believed that the weakening of the desire to procreate was caused by the progress of civilization and attributed the reduction in family size to the individual's ambitions to improve his position in society. Using a comparison, he argued that just as water can rise only under the force of capillarity in thin tubes, an individual can rise in the social scale only by having fewer children. The development of individualism and the desire for personal improvement and that of the children in advanced societies created, in his view, a state of mind conducive to declining fertility (Dumont, 1890). While agreeing that changes in social environment due to the progress of civilization were at the basis of the fertility decline, other writers (Hankins, 1930) attributed the latter more to the diversion of energies from procreation to the intellectual and physical activities imposed by the way of life. The declining birth rate then was supposed to reflect the pressure of those needs". (U.N., 1973: 154-55).

Demographic Transition

Although Landry was the first to postulate the theory of demographic transition as early as in 1909, it was further elaborated lucidly by a famous sociologist Notestein (1945). According to him ".....the growth of Europe in the modern era involved initially declining mortality produced by the process of modernization as a whole, including rising levels of living and new controls over disease. Fertility responded more slowly to modernization, but ultimately began a decline through the widespread use of contraception under the impact of such factors as growing individualism and rising levels of aspiration developed in urban industrial living." Noting that the more rapid response of mortality than of fertility to the forces of modernization was probably inevitable, he distinguished three types or stages of demographic evolution.

a. Population with incipient decline or "transition completed" (United States, Europe, Australia), characterised by a fertility rate declining to or even below the replacement level;
b. A transitional type of population (Soviet Union, Japan, some countries in Latin America) with a rate of growth which is still relatively rapid, but where a decline in the birth rate is well established; and
c. Population with high growth potentials or transitional growth not yet begun (most of the countries in Africa, Asia and latin America), where fertility remains high with no tendency to decline and where the high, but declining death rate is the main growth factor. He was of the opinion that the study of the beginning of economic development and demographic transition in certain non-European countries suggested that the principles drawn from the European demographic transition would be widely applicable in the world.

Theory of Multibasic Response

Kingsley Davis gave yet another addition to the theory on demographic transition on the following lines. "Although generally overlooked because of our pre-occupation with the contraceptive issue, the fact is that every country in north-west Europe reached to its persistent excess of births over deaths with virtually the entire range of possible responses. Regardless of nationality, language and religion, each industrialising nation tended to postpone marriage, to increase celibacy, to resort to abortion, to practice contraception in some form, and to emigrate overseas. The timing and relative importance of the reactions were not identical in the various countries, and of course methods could not be used that were not then technically feasible for the public at large (e.g. harmless sterilization); but the remarkable thing is that all of the north-west European countries reacted, that they did so in each case with the reappearance of the whole range of responses and that virtually the entire panorama was later repeated in Japan" (Davis, 1963: 350-51). He further elaborated: "My own view is that no society has been geared to a sustained high rate of national increase except by conquest. Under a prolonged drop in mortality with industrialization, people in North-West Europe and Japan found that their accustomed demographic behaviour was handicapping them in their effort to take advantage of the opportunities being provided by the emerging economy. They accordingly began changing their behaviour. Thus, it was in a sense the rising prosperity itself, viewed from the stand point of the individual's desire to get ahead and appear respectable, that forced a modification of his reproductive behaviour.

Mortality decline impinged on the individual by enlarging his family. Unless something were done to offset this effect, it gave him, as a child, more siblings with whom to share whatever derived from his parents as well as more likelihood of reckoning with his parents for a longer period of life; and, as an adult, it gave him a more fragmented and more delayed share of the patrimony with which to get married and found his own family, while at the same time it saddled him, in founding the family with the task of providing for more children for rearing them, educating them, endowing their marriages, etc., in a manner assuring them a status no lower than his .... The parent neèded to conserve some means for himself, because of longer life-expectancy and because of the importance of capital for seizing opportunities or staving off disaster in the fluid situation of the times" (Davis, 1963: 352).

These are some of the major general theories on population postulated by sociologists and other related social scientists. A few theories related to various specific dimensions of population studies are being highlighted below.

Theories on Fertility

Intermediate Variables

Although the pioneering work on determinants of human fertility was undertaken by Lorimer, an anthropologist, a systematic and exhaustive classification of the determinants of fertility behaviour was originally presented by Kingsley Davis and Judith Blake through their epoch making contribution in the field of fertility behaviour, "Social structure and Fertility: An Analytic Framework", which was originally published in 1956 in the Journal on 'Economic Development and Cultural Change'. Subsequently it was reproduced by Charls B. Nam in 'Population and Society' and in several other books and periodicals. It is a classical piece of work for studying fertility behaviour whether among the low or high fertility communities or the countries. A brief mention of its salient features would be highly relevant here in view of its great contribution to revolutionising fertility research all over the world. The authors have classified all the prominent determinants of fertility behaviour under three broad categories, designated as "Intermediate Variables". The first category of intermediate variables is known as "Intercourse Variables"; the second category as "Conception Variables" and the last category "Gestation Variables". Several specific variables associated with these stages of the life cycle of family formation have been identified and elaborated in this framework. Although, this framework would cover most of the determinants of high and low fertility behaviour, certain omissions in it have been identified by subsequent researchers.

Freedman's Conceptual Model

Ronald Freedman (1975) operationalised the intermediate variables into a conceptual model for facilitating empirical research in the field of fertility behaviour. In addition to specifying the position and the nature of casual relationships of various intermediate variables in the conceptual model, he also added the new and promising concept of 'family size norm' as a synonym for fertility behaviour at the attitudinal level. It can be used as a fertility variable for predicting the future fertility of un-wed mothers and mothers whose fertility formation has not been completed. The joint contribution of Davis and Blake along with that of Ronald Freedman together made the fertility research more precise and scientific. In fact, their combined contributions gave a depth of content and meaning to the theory on fertility.

The Freedman's conceptual model has been further elaborated and updated recently by Ruth Simmons, et al., (1983) and similarly the concept of intermediate variables of Davis and Blake was also given further elaboration by Bongaarts and Potter (1983) by giving it the new name of "Proximate determinants or fertility", wherein they identified certain high priority determinants of fertility behaviour, which together explain the largest proportion of variations in fertility behaviour in the particular population they have studied. According to them the 'Proximate Variables' are: age at first marriage, the use of contraception, breastfeeding, post-partum amenorrhea, birth interval and induced abortion.

Value of Children

The concept of value of children became yet another major additional determinants of fertility behaviour during the recent past. It is a multi-dimensional and multi-disciplinary concept. Its various dimensions have roots in several disciplines of social sciences including economics, sociology, anthropology and psychology. Economists, notably Becker (1960), Easterlin (1969), Leibenstein (1957) and Robinson and Horlacher (1971) expanded and empirically studied various aspects of value of children in the name of satisfaction (Benefits) and cost of children as an economic dimension of value of children. In addition to these 'pioneers' many other economists also studied this problem in different countries.

Sociologists and anthropologists have also made distinct and decisive contribution in identifying various dimensions of value of children from the view point of 'Culture and Society'. In this context the most important pioneering work was done by a team of interdisciplinary social demographers on "The value of children : A Cross-national study" carried out in the Asian context (Arnold, et al., 1975). Subsequently many other sociologists and anthropologists have studied this problem on a cross-national and also within a sub-cultural basis in different countries (Nag, et al., 1978; Mahadevan, 1979). In a recent nation-wide study on 'Determinants of Fertility Behaviour' conducted in India, Mahadevan (1985-1987) has identified several dimensions of value of children as the principal determinants of fertility behaviour compared to all other factors, which was confirmed through path analysis. Its importance was relatively less in Kerala, where matrilineal legacy of the population slightly diminished the importance of value of sons as compared to other determinants of fertility behaviour. Through this study and another in-depth study (Mahadevan and Sumangala, 1987) conducted on a comparative basis between Kerala and Andhra in India, further discovered the significance of studying the value of children in relation to the first son, second son and so on. The later study confirms that in future more emphasis has to be given for studying the importance given to the second son or more sons rather than studying the importance attached to first sons. The reason for this is the universal desire for at least one son. The desire for a second son is not uniform and general and is specific to different communities, cultural groups and also depending on the variety of other determinants including the risk involved in the life of the first son, risk associated with old age security and so on. Therefore, the concept of value of children emerged as one of the most promising areas of further study dealing with fertility behaviour.

Wealth flow Theory

Another social scientist, Caldwell (1976), while disagreeing with the theory on demographic transition stated that most of the premises of this theory are not relevant every where. Therefore, he postulated an alternative theory based on the experience gained from the tribal society of Africa. His theory may have greater application in selected tribal communities and peasant Societies, but it may not be fully applicable universally.

The salient aspects of his theory stated as follows: "In general, in societies of every type and stage of development, fertility behaviour is rational. . . whether high or low fertility is economically rational is determined. . . by the direction of the inter-generational wealth flow. This flow has been from younger to older generations in all traditional societies; and it is apparently impossible... for a reversal... to occur before the family is largely nucleated....

From the demographic view point, the most important social experts (from Western Europe) have been the concept of the predominance of the nuclear family with its strong conjugal tie and the concept of concentrating concern and expenditure on one's children. The latter does not automatically follow from the former, although it is likely to follow continuing Westernization; but the latter must be preceded by the former. There probably is no close relationship in timing between economic modernization and fertility .... Family nucleation and the reversal of the inter-generational wealth flow are likely to penetrate deeply into the Third World in the next half century, almost independently of the success of industrialization, and almost inevitably, they will guarantee slower global population growth" (pp. 355-356). Caldwell, has given the major features of generational changes and wealth flow in the following lines.

Generation: "In some traditional societies the older generations (within the family) may merely consist of parents and possibly grand parents, as well as parents-in-law; in others, uncles, aunts, and even great uncles or older cousins may play a role. Sometimes - and admittedly this places some strain on a strictly inter-generational approach - a rather similar role may be played by older siblings or even siblings of the opposite sex (or occasionally siblings with greater education or power in the new society). In many societies the relation of wives to their husbands is similar to that of children to fathers..." (Caldwell, 1982: 173-174).

Wealth: "This includes all sort of goods, services, and guarantees or power to command these. Examples are (1) the ability of a mother-in-law to order about her daughter-in-law even if it does not make house-keeping more efficient, and (2) guarantees of help in years of scarcity and devastation, of assistance if one's neighbour raises his hand against one... of support in old age ...."(Caldwell, 1982; 174). While critically discussing his theory Namboodiri (1986) has identified three major propositions which can be empirically tested for the validity of this theory in a given population. They are: (i) only if the family becomes nucleated will fertility drop, (ii) industrialization is not a necessary condition for fertility decline; and (iii) fertility decline starts with the reversal of the direction of inter-generational "wealth flow", which in all traditional societies has been from the younger to the older generation.

Structural Change and Fertility

Adnan (1982) from Bangladesh has developed a theoretical basis bringing about certain structural changes in certain strata of society for the control of fertility. It is based on the assumption that fertility is high in the lower strata of society and low in the higher strata of society. According to his thesis, structural changes have to be studied based on detailed system of stratification. This theoretical basis is expressed in the following lines: "Survival mediated through patronage is likely to provide employment for all employable members of the loyal household or none. The increased generation of labour power within the household will be thus encouraged by the consideration of obtaining the maximum share of whatever patronage is available, if and when it is provided. No anti-nationalist pressure would exist on these counts" (Adnan, 1979: 105). The same view was expressed by McNicoll (1982) in his similar theoretical postulation.

Normative Approach

This theoretical basis was postulated by Ryder. He wrote: "Human society regulates the behaviour of members, through norms... The individual acquires norms through indoctrination" (Ryder, 1979: 198). Applying this general proposition to reproductive behaviour "Each reproductive act may be thought of as an implicit contract. In making a decision to have a baby, the costs and benefits perceived depend on the terms of that contract, because it spells out the rights and responsibilities of the parties involved, (e.g., parents and children). The contract exists because the occurrence of a child is consequential to others beyond the immediate decision makers, and those others are prepared to administer rewards and punishments to insure that the individual decisions correspond with the collective will" (Ryder, 1980: 198). Ryders normative approach emphasises the social pattern underlying the idea of family formation.

Social Development, Cultural Change and Fertility Decline

It is the latest of the series of contributions made to study particularly the declining fertility of a given population. This author (Mahadevan, 1987) has formulated a new conceptual model for the study of the determinants of fertility decline based on his study of a successful low fertility region in India viz., Kerala state. It is the first of this kind for studying fertility decline. This model could also be used for studying general fertility behaviour. There are many specific new features noticed in this model compared to the existing ones. A number of propositions can be gleaned out of this model for testing any given population. Fertility changes may occur under the following situations viz., (1) When government and/or voluntary agencies directly and efficiently promote certain interventions to control fertility, it may lead to decline in fertility; (2) Economic development is not an essential condition for fertility decline, though it may also contribute to decline in nuptiality. (3) Favourable ecological and cultural changes are needed to facilitate the fertility change; (4) Creation of necessary infrastructural facilities on several fronts enables the rapid diffusion of contraceptions leading to decline in fertility; (5) Developments aimed at improving the quality of life of a cross section of population including: (a) children; (b) eligible couple and women in particular; (c) old population etc., are necessary for the fall in fertility; (6) An expanded and efficient family planning programme integrated with MCH and other health programme may lead to decline in fertility; (7) Increase in cost of living including opportunity cost contributes to reduction in fertility; (8) Modernization in several aspects of life is needed for the normal decline in fertility; (9) Several kinship and other social obligations born out of cultural patterns and their existence may also lead to differences in fertility behaviour. All these may contribute to certain structural changes in specific dimensions of a society viz., individual, social, cultural and developmental fields which together facilitate the decline in mortality followed by fall in fertility. The preceding structural changes, services policies, and programmes may contribute to individual level behavioural change leading to changes in fertility and the quality of life. Some of the behavioural attributes are also equally important to regulate the fertility. A number of propositions can also be formulated based on such concepts that are given in this model. These concepts may include the changes in norms and values, value of children, family size norm, old age security, child labour and norms about intermediate variables. In addition to these social dimensions of behavioural change certain psychological factors such as changes in attitude, motivation, perception, anxiety and fear, several intermediate variables and patterns of decision-making are equally important for different levels of fertility change. Over and above these changes, the influence of one or more intermediate variables for example age at marriage could also lead to changes in fertility and improvement in the quality of life. But changes in age at marriage cannot take place in isolation without certain structural changes in the society. It is equally true for acceptance of contraception. Unlike other models it gives equal importance to fertility change along with difference in the quality of life. Further, this model places equal emphasis on social development along with certain essential cultural change for achieving fertility decline and improving the quality of life. The social development conceived here is different from the model advocated by conventional economists. Not much importance is given here for improvement in per capita income. Instead expansion of infrastructural facilities, provision of minimum needs and such other welfare schemes, improvement in nutritional status, availability and utilization of health and family planning services, improvement in environmental conditions, expansion of educational facilities and rapid increase in literacy level followed by the decline in child mortality etc. With the active efforts and intervention of appropriate programme mixes by the government and voluntary agencies are given importance. The desirable cultural change may cover the changes in value of son preference, improvement in status of women, individual and social modernization, including better facilities and life style. Thus, all these aspects can be classified under overall social development and cultural change resulting into fertility decline and improvement in the quality of life of the population in general. This theoretical assumption is very close to the reality of population change in the context of changing socio-cultural and population scenario in several progressive developing countries viz., Kerala, Sri Lanka and such other regions in Asia, Latin America and even in Africa.

Sociology and Family Planning

Although several factors that influence fertility may have influence on family planning, the later has been studied separately from fertility behaviour. It is done because there are certain exclusive factors which are important to understand family planning behaviour. Further, family planning is more a sensitive behavioural issue than fertility per se. Under family planning aspects issues like communication, education, service and follow-up, incentives and several other interventions have greater influence than even some of the other common determinants of fertility. For one reason or the another not much advance could be made so far in theorising any aspects of family planning. But certain piecemeal efforts have been made in relation to decision making and family planning, communication and family planning, adoption process and family planning, patterns and process of communication and their credibility in family planning behaviour. Efforts have also been made in relation to rumour and in the role of incentives in acceptance or rejection of the family planning methods. Among these contributions, a few which may fall within the purview of sociology have been highlighted here.

Social Development, Cultural Change and Fertility Decline: A Model

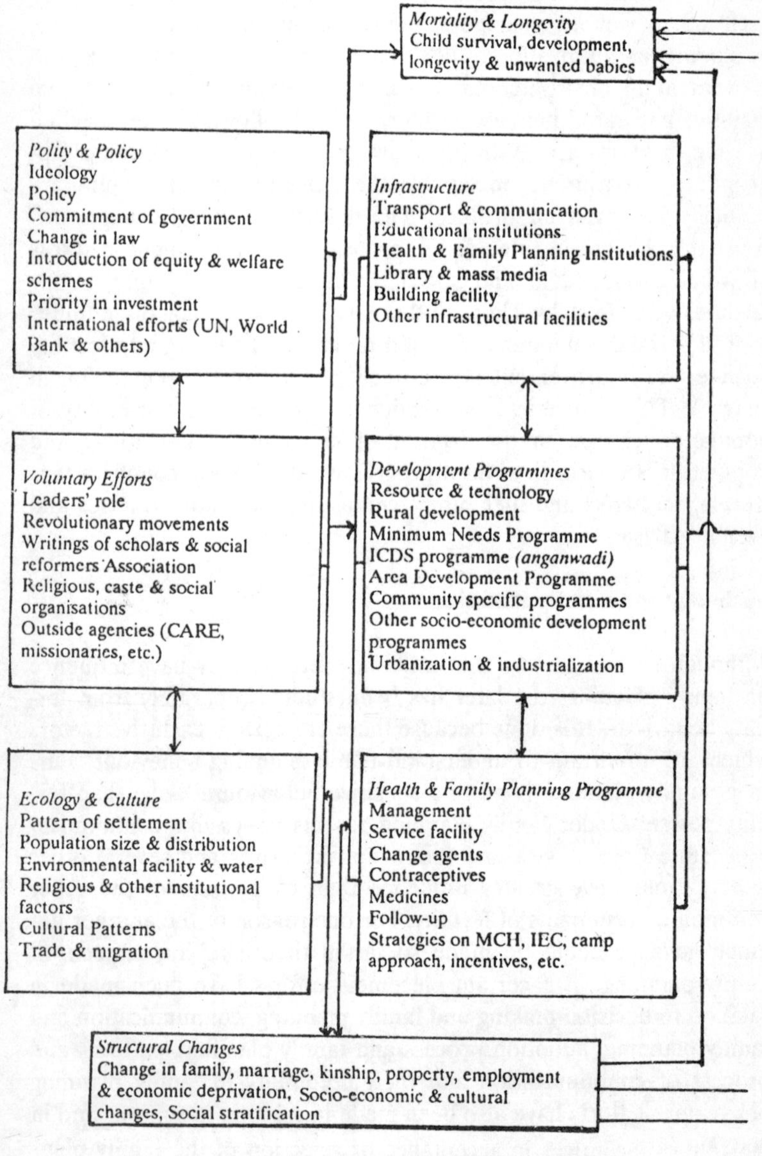

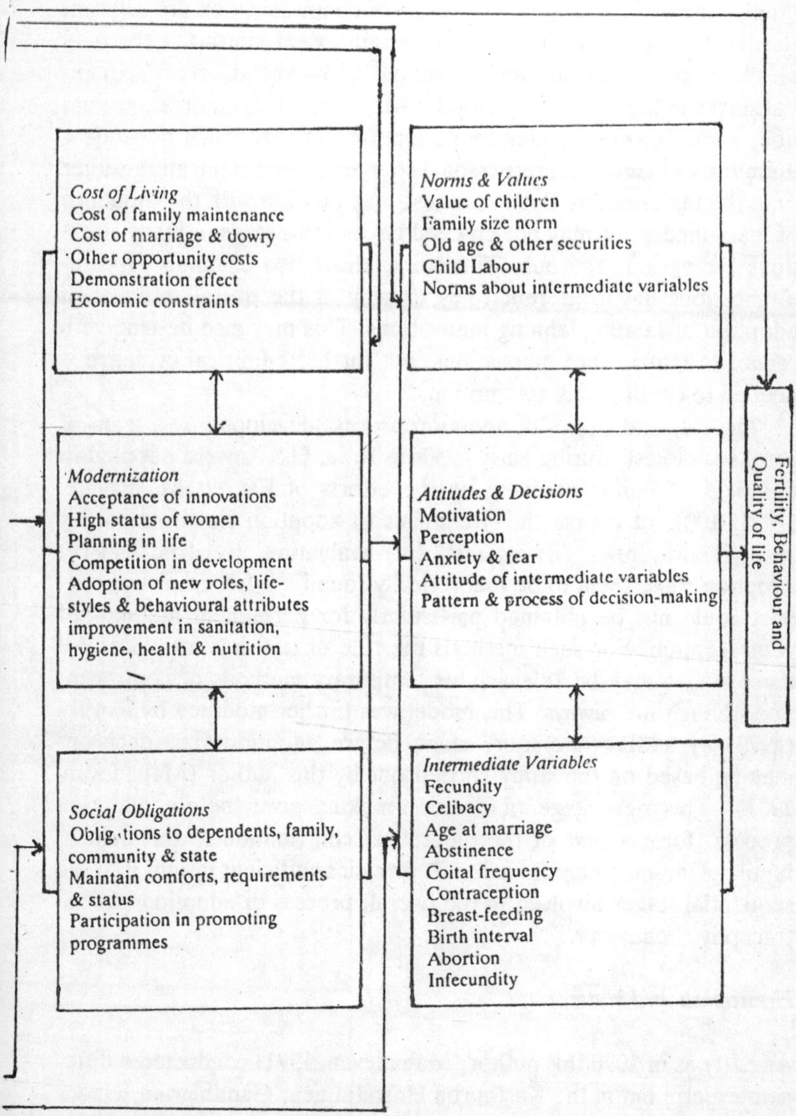
Cost of Living
Cost of family maintenance
Cost of marriage & dowry
Other opportunity costs
Demonstration effect
Economic constraints
Norms & Values
Value of children
Family size norm
Old age & other securities
Child Labour
Norms about intermediate variables
Modernization
Acceptance of innovations
High status of women
Planning in life
Competition in development
Adoption of new roles, life-styles & behavioural attributes
improvement in sanitation, hygiene, health & nutrition
Attitudes & Decisions
Motivation
Perception
Anxiety & fear
Attitude of intermediate variables
Pattern & process of decision-making
Fertility, Behaviour and Quality of life
Social Obligations
Obligations to dependents, family, community & state
Maintain comforts, requirements & status
Participation in promoting programmes
Intermediate Variables
Fecundity
Celibacy
Age at marriage
Abstinence
Coital frequency
Contraception
Breast-feeding
Birth interval
Abortion
Infecundity

Communication and Contraception

It has been fairly confirmed that both inter personal sources of communication and mass-media channels of communication are relevant for developing awareness and to a certain extent interest in the field of adoption process on family planning. However, different sequential stages in the process of adoption viz., awareness, interest, evaluation, trial, decision-making and adoption are very much dependent upon the influence of interpersonal sources of communication rather than the mass-media. But awareness may develop with the influence of mass-media but may not proceed beyond this stage in many situations for various reasons. Therefore, these two channels of communications have different roles to play in the overall process of adoption of family planning innovations. This may also be true with regard to many other innovations, but further empirical evidence is needed to confirm this assumption.

The classical stages of adoption process developed by a team of rural sociologists during early 1950s in Iowa, U.S.A. were adopted in the field of family planning by the efforts of Everett M. Rogers (1971: 100), of course the five stages of adoption classified earlier viz., (i) awareness, (ii) interest, (iii) evaluation, (iv) trial and (v) adoption stage seem to be theoretically sound but full empirical support could not be obtained particularly for permanent methods of contraception. For such methods the role of trial has no place. All these stages may be relevant for temporary methods of contraception, though not always. This model was further modified by Rogers (1973) by adding one more stage before adoption viz., decision-making based on the study carried out by this author (Mahadevan, 1971). This new stage of decision-making given before adoption process, form a part of the theoretical contribution to the field of family planning communication. It provides sufficient insight into the sequential stages involved in the overall process of adoption of contraceptive behaviour.

Homophili and Heterophili

As early as in 1970 this author (Mahadevan, 1971) conducted a diffusion experiment at the Kasthurba Hospital near Gandhigram. Under this experiment all the women who received maternity service from the Kasthurba hospital were given a set of identity cards of the hospital and were advised to pass them, on to people whom they liked in their village after the treatment. Based on the characteristics of these clients with those of the people, who received the cards, an analysis of the flow of communication was carried out. A prominent and promising idea emerged from the analysis was that a pattern existed in the process of communication between the communicator and the communicatee. This pattern was identified and named as "Similar" and "Dissimilar" pattern of communication with regard to various socio-demographic characteristics of these communicators and communicatees. Out of the several characteristics studied, a definite pattern emerged with regard to the religion and caste characteristics of these two groups. In other words, by and large, people belonging to the same caste and religion communicated with people from similar backgrounds. Although this author had coined the term of similar and dissimilar patterns of communication, subsequently Rogers (1973) gave different nomenclature to the same and called them 'homophilous' (same) and 'heterophilous' (dissimilar) patterns of communication. In the former category of communication the communicator and communicatee have more or less certain similar characteristics, but those in the latter pattern do not. The pattern of communication is also conditioned by the type of credibility - competence and safety credibility - manifests by the communicator to the communicatee. This concept has emerged as a major theoretical basis in the field of family planning communication.

Satisfied Adopters, Credibility and Diffusion

Satisfied family planning adopters are found to be one of the most credible personal channels of communication noticed, so far, in this field of family planning research. It is but natural that a closely known satisfied adopter from the neighbourhood of a client, who also has certain other social links as friend or neighbour or relative, can provide the much needed credibility to an eligible couple who generally suffer from anxiety and fear for the adoption of family planning. It was found that 80 per cent of the eligible couples manifested certain degrees of anxiety and fear (Mahadevan, 1984) they may not adopt family planning unless a credible source comes forward to alleviate their fear and anxiety. This idea was confirmed through a series of investigations carried out on satisfied adopters of family planning by this author (Mahadevan 1967, 68, 73, 74a and 76b and 1984). When a quasi-experimental study was carried out in a group meeting situation in the field area facilitating interaction between satisfied adopters and non-adopters, it was confirmed that after frequent exchange of information between satisfied adopters and non-adopters a significant increase in credibility and adoption of family planning among the non-adopters could be observed (Mahadevan, 1984: 76). Therefore, it is confirmed beyond any doubt that frequent interaction made between satisfied adopters and non-adopters would lead to favourable behavioural change leading to adoption of family planning among the rural population. This theoretical findings validate the existing high degree of credibility attached to the satisfied adopters for alleviating the fear and anxiety on the part of clients about family planning and subsequently for motivating them to accept family planning.

Decision-making in Family Planning

Decision-making for acceptance or non-acceptance of family planning forms yet another major theoretical field for understanding and predicting the future contraceptive behaviour. This author through a series of two continuous studies on decision-making has developed a number of new concepts besides developing a theory on decision-making itself. He has identified a number of dimensions for the abstract concept of decision-making. They were identified on the basis of a number of case studies, exploratory studies and surveys conducted in this field of study. He could analytically conceptualise the role of communication in general, intraspouse communication in particular and a number of sources of communication as important area of influence in decision-making. Even the extent of knowledge possessed by the client could influence the decision in favour or against or remain indecisive. Several other barriers and facilitating factors that influence the course of decision-making were also identified. Time-lag was yet another dimension of decision-making. Over and above these factors, the concept of decision-making itself has been classified trichotomously into: (i) decided in favour of (ii) decided against and (iii) undecided for empirical viability. Such a classification would provide feasibility for studying this abstract concept in future also.

For giving conceptual clarity he has developed a number of decisiogram in which he has suitably depicted the interaction of personal and impersonal sources of communication with the clients, their positive and negative influence on the eligible couple besides showing the direct and indirect influence of several forces on the couples who makes decisions in favour of or against family planning. Added to this, a systems of model on decision-making has also been evolved, which provides a holistic understanding of the influence of various factors during the entire process of decision-making. These conceptual refinement was possible through a feasible operational definition that he contributed on decision-making . . . "the decision in favour of or against adoption of contraception is invariably a resultant of the interaction and influence of both personal and/or impersonal, favourable or unfavourable forces or both, occurring over a period of time" (1984. 30) There are a few more such isolated formulations of theoretical basis in the field of family planning, but paucity of time and space do not allow for the present author to proceed further.

Sociology and Mortality

Although the field of research on mortality under population studies provides immense scope for sociologists, anthropologists and other social scientists in the field of research, render service and promote health programmes in different ways, it has been the least area out of several dimensions of population studies, where social scientists who has been engaged, so far, in performing one or the other role in population studies. It was largely because of the assumption that the study of mortality is a medical field and further perceived that it is an area where only statistically dominated population scientists alone could do effective work. It was caused by the present day involvement of medical as well as statistically oriented demographers largely working in this field. Of course, the medical people continue to work in the field of death and statisticians repeat the same research on life tables and other model building activities. But they have not gone beyond this frontiers of research. When we make retrospective content analysis of seminars, symposia, workshops etc., that were carried out by the I.U.S.S.P, W.H.O., UNICEF etc., till the beginning of the 1980's it would reveals that only a narrow area of mortality was repeatedly taken up for study by medical personal and statistically oriented demographers, had not realised the expanded scope of study under mortality because of the absence of comprehensive framework and conceptual model. Therefore, it was a misnomer on their part as well as on the part of social scientists to believe that whatever research and programme interventions carried out hitherto were sufficient in the field of mortality studies.

It was from 1984 onwards that a rethinking started on expanding the scope of the studies on mortality and led to the promotion of programme in this field based on a theoretical-cum-methodological contributions made particularly by three authors viz., Hentry Mosley and Lincoln Chen (1983) and Mahadevan (1983 and 1984) which made several scholars to realise the wide scope for expanding their activities and involving the social scientists in a big way. While the former two scholars gave greater emphasis to medical and less emphasis to other determinants of mortality, this author provided emphasis to a large number of interdisciplinary category of "Life Affecting Variables". Of course their relevance and priority of importance may have to be identified through future studies. The most comprehensive work in this direction was made by the third author through his innovative and valuable work on "Mortality, Biology and Society: An Analytical Framework and Conceptual Model" which made a sudden drift, expansion and diversification of research and other activities, in this field besides large scale involvement of social scientists in this field. This model generated interest and provided knowledge among other social scientists to attempt and develop small-scale models also for developing countries based on their professional background and interest besides diversifying the scope of activities under the field of mortality studies. The diversification in themes considered under the field of mortality for different types of academic meetings by IUSSP from 1984 onwards is a testimony of the impact of the above framework made at the international level. The outstanding unique features of this model are the following: it provides a comprehensive logically related a dozen list of variables with several sub-variables under each one of them; gave a most appropriate nomenclature viz., Life Affecting Variables (LVS) to refer to all the determinants of mortality; provided all the salient factors under a wide spectrum of social, cultural, ecological and many other types of factors that are relevant and neglected hitherto under mortality studies and gave an appropriate conceptual model to study the nature of causal relationship of the variables. This framework and the conceptual model together may revolutionise studies in the near future as happened in the case of fertility studies by the contributions of Davis and Blake and Ronald Freedman. Therefore, from now onwards sociologists and other social scientists may involve themselves in greater number to carry out studies and other activities in this sub-area of population studies.

Migration and Urbanisation

These two areas of population studies have already become a major field of research activity of social scientists all over the world. Since several decades sociologists have been working in a big way for the study of urbanization and migration, this can evidently be seen in most of the sociology text books that have been produced during the last 50 or more years. Long before the demographers identified this area the sociologists have been studying urbanization and migration as an integral part of their profession. They continue to do so even now. They are also being chosen as policy makers and advisors besides researchers for developing urban areas all over the world. Similar is the case with regard to migration also. The sociologists, compared to many other professionals have acquired a pre-eminent position in the study of urbanization and migration. Since, this fact is now well-known, there is no need here to elaborate the major role of sociologists under this area.

Population Education

Population education again constitute a major field of work for the population sociologists. In many countries mostly sociologists, psychologists, social workers, and other social scientists continue to work in this field in a big way. Since population education has to be carried on among the different categories of family members viz., parents, eligible couples, adolescent children and children below the age of fourteen, besides school going children and dropped out children, only social scientists can do full justice to the promotion of population education among these diverse categories of population in a society. Based on this reality the concepts of population studies relevant to different segment of population have been carried forward by sociologists for the promotion of population control programme. It can be justified further, when we examine the definition of population education given by UNESCO and the role that sociologists could play in translating this definition into actual practice. The UNESCO (1970) defined population education in the following lines "Population Education is an educational programme which provides for a study of the population education in the family, community, nation and world with the purpose of developing in the students, rational and responsible attitudes and behaviour towards coping with the situation."

Status of Women

Raising status of women is a major developmental strategy on the lines of social betterment, which may be feasible and less expensive than the economic models of development followed for improving the quality of population in general. The experience of Kerala, Sri Lanka and several other progressive developing countries of Asia have confirmed that, social development particularly the emancipation of women has several multiplying benefits on different dimensions of development. Even the social development has been accelerating at a lesser cost and on a quicker basis by emancipating women. It showed tremendous improvement in the quality of life in general and particularly fast reduction in all forms of human wastages (Mortality), early and quick acceptance of family planning, rapid reduction in fertility and all-round improvement in the life of the population as a whole. Under this assumption only improvement in status of women may have to be considered as a feasible theoretical proposition for population stabilization.

The concept of status has been conceived differently by different authors. "Linton (1936: 113) defined the status as the place of an individual in society and that it is a 'Collection of rights and duties', with certain roles to put them (right and duties) into action." In modern social science, "Status denotes (a) position in a social system, involving reciprocal expectation of action with respect to occupants of other positions in the same structure, (b) place with respect to the distribution of prestige within a social system, and sometimes, by implications, with respect to the distribution of rights, obligations, power and authority within the same system as in the phrases, 'high status', and 'low status'; (c) high place with respect to the distribution of rights, obligations, power and authority within the same system as in the phrases, 'Status keeper'" (Encyclopaedia of Social Sciences, 1934: 373).

The status of women in the real and complete sense is a recent and emerging concept, though women in general enjoyed certain privileges, positions, rights, duties, roles, power and authority in varying degrees in different societies. However, they did not enjoy equal and extensive status in society as in the case of men. The concept of status of women has been defined by a few scholars giving different emphasis to its specific dimensions. The term status is used, first, as an access to resources such as education, gainful employment, and health services and, second, the position (Power, Prestige, Authority) that a woman has in various situations. The term "role" refers to the various activities that a woman performs in relation to her status in a given situation (Oppong, 1980 and Dixon, 1978). Another author differentiates between power and the status of women. While defining he states the term "women's power can be distinguished from women's status, in that status refers to women's overall position in the society, while power refers to women's ability to influence and control at the interpersonal level. Thus, female power can be defined as women's ability to control or change other women's or men's behaviour and the ability to determine important events in their lives, even when men and older women are opposed to them" (Safilios - Rothschild, 1982: 117). Thus, the status of women like the general concept of status, is a multi-dimensional and dynamic one which is considered on a relative basis. It comprises several dimensions like one's own legacy and achievements including money, materials, merits and privileges and the autonomy to take one's own decisions. Along with such roles, progressive characteristics and achievements go together to manifest the status. All these dimensions of status may have value over a particular period of time, with reference to a situation, and may be able to function on their own lines.

On the basis of the above notions of the concept of women, a theoretical basis for the study and developing status for the women were evolved by this author. This theoretical contribution has several advantages for policy formulation and undertaking sound studies on fertility, mortality, family planning, migration etc., in relation to the status of women. It is the first conceptual model and analytical framework developed on status of women linking with population parameters. This analytical framework is very comprehensive and consists of a universal list of 18 categories of variables and their sub-variables. Since, the approach of this theoretical formulation is on a global basis appropriate and suitable, factors from this framework can be considered based on the need for the population under study. However, the conceptual model based on this analytical framework (Status affecting variables) provide a sound basis for visualizing the probable causal relationship in an empirical situation. It is needed in any high quality research and for deeper understanding of the problem in relation to different population parameters. The details of this contribution is given in a forthcoming book of this author

(Mahadevan, 1989). This aspect of social development is a high priority area for rapid development of fertility control programme in a feasible and economically viable basis in developing countries. Sociologists and other social scientists have a great role to play in applying this model for faster development of society and population stabilization in less affluent developing countries.

The scope for sociologists and other social scientists to work in the field of Population Studies is immense. In this context it has to be particularly pointed out that there is greater scope also for them to work in the fields of population policy formulations and promotion of population control programme; these areas have tremendous potentiality for the successful participation of Sociologists. The author's forthcoming book on "Fertility Policies in Asian Countries" (Mahadevan, 1989) tries to highlight the possible role of Sociologists in helping the government in formulating, improving and expanding population policy based on the demographic situation, and diversity of development in different countries.

Uniqueness of this Study

This book on "Religion, Social Change and Fertility Behaviour", based on a study carried out in the Travancore region of Kerala is a fascinating and excellent piece of contribution for several reasons. First of all, any meaningful study carried out in Kerala on demographic aspects will be interesting because Kerala holds a unique position in the world of demographic literature. The experience of rapid decline of fertility and mortality in Kerala without appreciable parallel or preceding economic improvement among the people is not common in any part of the world. Even without optimum economic development, Kerala has attained a very high degree of other kinds of social developments. This reality has questioned the hitherto accepted assumption that economic development is a major pre-condition for the decline in mortality and fertility. But Kerala's experience has disproved it. It is not Kerala alone shown this deviation even Sri Lanka also has manifested more or less a similar scenario. Therefore, this study of Kerala is an illuminating piece of information.

Since, the demographic studies have very rarely considered religion and caste as major social stratification variables, we were in darkness and could not know how fertility behaviour differentially manifested across these major cultural groups. Although, most of the societies in developing countries are stratified with such factors, it is highly realistic and relevant to consider this factor along with the study of fertility and other demographic parameters. This uniqueness is seen in the present study, which may form a pacesetter for similar sound studies to be taken up in future in other parts of the country and outside. Further, the methodology applied in this study is both unique and appropriate because it shows how various independent variables influence fertility among different cultural groups, both young and old population. Moreover, the application of path analysis for finding out the relative influence of each major independent variable on fertility separately among different cultural groups provide scope for appropriate generalization leading to theoretical development and also for providing ideas for judicious selection of inputs among the low and high fertility communities on the basis of their determinants of fertility behaviour for ultimate population stabilization. These are only a few salient specialities of this valuable piece of work.

The present book comprises nine chapters. It begins with a general account of social change and differential fertility, that have taken place in the Travancore region, followed by the presentation of data under the captions on nuptiality and fertility, socio-economic status and fertility, value of children, breastfeeding, birth interval, contraception, path analysis, and it ends with the summary of the findings and their implications. The dependent variable of the study is the live births, and all other variables referred to earlier constitute the independent variables. Religion and duration of married life of women have been kept as control variables throughout the analysis.

The opening chapter focuses attention on a macro basis about the people, their religious diversity, changes in various aspects of their life style and culture including the social change in general and also their existing differential fertility. While discussing these aspects, their past and present position with respect to most of the features have been covered on a comprehensive and comparative basis in order to give a realistic view of their differences, in culture, development and demographic dimensions. This chapter offers a fairly extensive coverage of social change in Kerala society as a backdrop to understand the relevance of studying this problem on a cross-cultural basis.

The second chapter deals with nuptiality and fertility; it discusses the age at marriage of wife and husband, the ideal age at marriage of girls and boys, the cost of marriage and determinants of age at marriage, such as education, occupation and income. The socio-economic status variables viz., family type, housing conditions, education, occupation, economic status and opportunity cost and their relation to the dependent variable have been studied in the third chapter. The fourth chapter concentrates on value of children, different dimensions of value of children, an index on value dimension and their relationship with fertility. Breastfeeding, postpartum amenorrhea and fertility across the three religious groups are presented in the fifth chapter, followed by birth intervals in the sixth chapter. The seventh chapter is on contraception and fertility, which include adoption and non-adoption of contraceptives and their effect on fertility, major determinants of family planning adoption status, viz., caste, education, income and occupation. The determinants of age at marriage and contraception have been specially considered here in view of their greater importance in explaining low fertility.

The findings of a path analysis are presented in the eighth chapter. Separate path analysis for the total population and the three religious groups, viz., Hindus, Christians and Muslims have also been carried out with the six selected major variables. The path diagram and path coefficients for each religion and for the total population are considered. In the last chapter the major findings of the present study have been summarised with suitable implications for policy formulations suggested. Thus, the present study attempts for the first time to explain the differential influence of the preceding list of demographic, developmental and cultural variables across different religious groups, which manifest differential fertility in a major region of Kerala state in India.

REFERENCES

Adnan, 1982: "Conceptualising Fertility Trends in Peripheral Foundation". In C. Hobn and R. Mackensen (Eds.). *Determinants of Fertility Trends: Major theories and new directions for research.* Ordina edition for the International Union for the Scientific Study of Population.

Arnold, F. & J.T. Fawcett, 1975: *The Value of Children* Vol. III, Honolulu, East-West Population Institute.

Becker Gary, S. 1960: "An Economic Analysis of Fertility". *In Demographic and Economic change in Developed Countries.* Universities National Bureau Committee for Economic Research, Special Conference Series, No. 11, Princeton University Press.

Bongaarts John & R.G., Potter, 1983: *Fertility, Biology and Behaviour : An Analysis of Proximate Determinants,* New York, Academic Press.

Caldwell, J. 1976: "Towards Restatement of Demographic Transition Theory". *Population and Development Review,* Vol. 2 pp. 321 - 366.

Caldwell, J. 1982: "Wealth flow Theory of Fertility Decline". In C. Hobn and R. Mackensen (Eds.). *Determinants of Fertility Trends: Major Theories and New Directions of Research.* Ordina Editions.

Davis, Kingsley & Judith Blake, 1968: "Social Structure and Fertility: An analytical

Framework" in *Population and Society*, Edt., Charles B. Nam pp. 196-215.

Dixon, Ruth, 1978: *Rural Women at work*, Baltimore: The Johns Hopkins University Press.

Dupreel, 1928: Deux assais sur le progre's part 3. Fromont, Demographic economique (1947), pp. 211. cited in "*The Determinants and Consequences of Population Trends*" Vol. I, U.N. 1973.

Durkheim, 1893: De la division du travail Social, 1960 ends pp. 237 - 244, 259 - 266 cited in "*The Determinants and Consequences of Population Trends*" Vol. I. U.N. 1973.

Easterlin, R. 1969: Towards a Socio-economic Theory of fertility. A survey of Recent Research on Economic factors in American Fertility, pp. 127 - 156 in S.J Behrman L. Corsa, Jr. and R. Freedman eds., *Fertility and Family Planning. A World view*, Ann Arbor, Mich. University of Michigan Press.

Freedman, Ronald, 1986: Theories of Fertility Decline: In *Fertility and Mortality*....edt., by K. Mahadevan, New Delhi, Sage Publications.

Freedman, Ronald, 1975: *The Sociology of Human Fertility: An Annotated Bibliography*, New York, Irwington Publication.

Freedman, Ronald: Pascal K. Whelpton & Arthee Campbell, 1959: *Family Planning, Sterility and Population Growth*, New York, McGraw Hill.

Hankins, 1930: "Does advancing civilization involve a decline in natural fertility", cited in "*The Determinants and Consequences of Population Trends*". Vol. I, U.N. 1973.

Linton, 1936: *The Study of Man*, New York, Appleton Century pp. 113-114 cited in *Encyclopaedia of Social Sciences*.

Landry, 1909: "Ees trois theories principles de la population" (1909, 1934 ed.); and his la revolution demographiq 1934. cited in "*The Determinants and Consequences of Population Trends*" Vol. I, U.N. 1973.

Leibenstein, Harvey, 1974: *The Economic Theory of Fertility*: Promising path or Blind alley, *JEL*, 12: 457 - 459.

Leibenstein, Harvey, 1957: *Economic Backwardness and Economic Growth*, New York, John Willy.

Mahadevan, K. 1988: *Population Dynamics in Indian States*, Vol. I & II, (Mimeo)

Mahadevan, K. 1989: *Fertility Policies in Asian Countries*, New Delhi, Sage Publications.

Mahadevan, K. & M. Sumangala 1987: *Social Development, Cultural Change and Fertility Decline: A study of Kerala's Fertility Change*, New Delhi, Sage Publications.

Mahadevan, K. 1986: *Fertility and Mortality: Theory, Methodology and Empirical Issues*; New Delhi, Sage Publications.

Mahadevan, K. 1984: *Decision-making and Diffusion in Family Planning*, Population Studies Centre, Tirupati, S.V. University.

Mahadevan, K. 1979: *Sociology of Fertility: Determinants of Fertility Differentials in South India*, New Delhi, Sterling Publishers.

Mahadevan, K. 1974: "Decision-making in a contraceptive Behaviour, A System approach", *Demography India*, Vol. 3, No. 2, Journal of the Association for the study of population, India.

Mahadevan, K. 1974: Determinants of non-contraception: An exploration in the process of decision-making among non-adopters, *Bulletin, The Gandhigram Institute of Rural Health and Family Planning*. Vol. IX. No. 2.

Mahadevan, K. Sethu and Govindachary, A. 1973: "Diffusion of Contraception": A hospital centred study on female sterilization, *Bulletin, The Gandhigram Institute of Rural Health and Family Planning*, Vol. VIII No. 1.

Mahadevan, K. 1968: "A Study of the decision - process in adoption of family planning methods". *Bulletin, The Gandhigram Institute of Rural Health and*

Family Planning, Vol. VI, No. 1.

Mahadevan, K. 1967: "Diffusion of Information". *Bulletin, Gandhigram Institute of Rural Health and Family Planning*, Vol. II, No. 3.

McNicoll, G. 1982: Institutional Determinants of Fertility Change. In C. John and R. Mackensen (Eds.). *Determinants of Fertility Trends: Major Theories and New Directions for Research.* Ordina edition.

Mougeolle, 1883: Statistique des civilizations. Cited in. *The Determinants and Consequences of Population Trends*" Vol. I, U.N. 1973.

Mosley, W.H. and Chen, Lincoln, C. 1984: An Analytical Framework for the study of Chiid survival in Developing Countries. In W.H. Mosley and Chen L.C. (Eds.) *Child Survival Strategies for Research. A supplement to Population and Development Review.* 10: 24-45 New York. The population council.

Nag, M., B.N.F, White and R.C. Peet, 1978: "An anthropological approach to the study of the economic value of children in Jawa and Nepal", *Current Anthropology,* Vol. 19, No. 2. pp. 293-306.

Nam, B. Charles (edt.), 1968: *Population and Society,* New York, The Florida State University.

Namboodiri, N.K. 1986: "Societal Development and Cultural Change, A Reappraisal of Selected theories" in *Fertility and Mortality...* edt. by K. Mahadevan, New Delhi, Sage Publications.

Namboodiri, N.K. 1960: *Fertility Differentials and Determinants in Kerala* (Mimeo).

Nitti 1984: Population and the Social System, Spengler, Der Untergang des Abendlandes (1921), Vol. 2 cited in. *'The Determinants and Consequences of Population Trends'*, Vol. I, U.N. 1973.

Notestein, 1945: "Population: the long view" his Economic problems of population change, (1953); and also his "The population of the World in the year 2000" (1956).

Oppong Christine, 1982: Familv Structure and Women's Reproduction and productive roles: Some conceptual and methodological of Issues, Anker Richard et al (ed.), *Women's Roles and Population Trends in the Third World,* London, Croom Helm.

Robinson, Warsen E., & David L. Horlacher 1971: *Population Growth and Economic Welfare,* Reports on population Family Planning, No. 6, New York: Population Council.

Rogers, M. Everett, 1973: *Communication Strategies for Family Planning*, New York, The Free Press.

Rogers, M. Everett, 1971: *Communication of Innovations : A Cross Cultural Approach.* New York, The Free Press.

Ruth, George, B. Simmons, Gayle, D. Ness & George B. Simmions, 1983: "On the Institutional Analysis of Populaticn Programmes", *Population and Development Review,* Vol. 9, No. 3.

Ryder, N.B., 1980: Where do babies come form, In H.M. Blalock (eds.), *Sociological theory and research. A Critical Appraisal.* New York. The Free Press.

Safilios Constantina - Rothschild 1982: Female power, Autonomy and Demographic change in the third World. Anker Richard et al (ed.), *Women's Roles and Population Trends in the third World,* London, Croom Helm, pp. 117-130.

U.N. 1973: *The Determinants and Consequences of Population Trend*, Vol. I & II, New York, pp. 33-63.

UNESCO 1970: "Regional Workshop on Population and Family Education Bangkok. Draft Final Report. UNESCO Regional office for Education in Asia, Bangkok.

Wilbert E. Moore, 1959: "Sociology and Demography" in *The Studies of Population : An Inventory and Appraisal* (Edt.) by Philip M. Hanser and Otis Dudley Duncan.

ONE

SOCIAL CHANGE AND DIFFERENTIAL FERTILITY

Kerala, a relatively small state, is located on India's South West Coast. The state of Kerala in the present form came into being on 1st November, 1956, under the States Re-organisation Act of 1956. This was formed by integrating the erstwhile Travancore, Cochin and Malabar states. It has an area of 38,863 sq. kms. It is 576 kms. long (North-south), while its breadth (West-East) ranges from 11 km. to 120 kms. The land has been divided into three ecological regions, viz., Coastal land, Midland and the Hilly regions. The two monsoons, South-West and North-East, give rains in Kerala making plenty of water available to the people of the state. Kerala's geography provides a partial explanation of its social structure and features; cultural complexity is generally an effect of geographical isolation. Kerala's political and cultural developments are conditioned to a large extent by these geographical and physical environments. According to Puthenkalam (1977) "Kerala is a land of contrasts. In the variegated picture of Kerala, social elements of yesterday and today and ways of life in centuries apart are found juxtaposed. A strong social ferment questioning the values held sacred for centuries is there, as well as a love for social values handed down from generation to generation."

Kerala differs generally from the rest of India in geography, land systems, crops and in customs and manners. Nature has given plenty of resources, but economically the state is at present one of the most hard-pressed, because of heavy population pressure. Kerala stands out as unique among the Indian states. It is one of the smaller states and has several unique characteristics; highest density of population, excess females over males in the total population, lower level of mortality and fertility, higher mean age at marriage among females, higher literacy rate, and higher proportion of workers in non-agricultural sector, when compared to other states in India. According to the 1981 census, the average density of population per square mile was 655 which is about three times higher than the all-India average; the literacy rate is 70.4 as against 36.2 in India. In the case of sex ratio, Kerala has 1,032 women for every thousand men as against 933 in India (Census, 1981). Hence, with respect to some of the demographic characteristics of its population, Kerala appears to be more akin to the developed societies of the west, whereas its economy is similar to that of a typical, developing nation of the east. These demographic changes have resulted concurrently with the other social changes that have taken place in the state.

Religion and Caste

In the field of religion and culture, Kerala presents a greater variety, in every phase of culture, from the most primitive to the most advanced. In clothing, food, and everyday habits of life, the people show a marked distinctiveness compared to the rest of India. Therefore, Kerala has been described as a living museum of ethnology, culture and religions, presenting every stage of development (Krishna Iyer, 1968). Kerala's religious system constitutes a "plurality of religions, and not only of religion as such, but also of plurality with each religion; its religious factor acting as a component of the culture of each of these groups. Hence, in Kerala, religion has really performed the function of providing social identity" (Neuve, 1983). the major religious groups are the Hindus, Christians and Muslims. According to the 1981 census, the Hindus constitute 58.2 per cent, Christians 20.6 and Muslims 21.2 per cent of the total population.

As regards religious tolerance, which is a manifestation of modernization, it is extensively noticed throughout the state, in both rural and urban areas. Religious institutions such as temples, churches and mosques have been established in very close proximity and function in a harmonious manner. The periodic and annual celebrations of religious functions of all the communities are more or less tolerated/celebrated together by other communities. Exchange of greetings and sharing of joy and feasts at religious functions take place among different sects which is very common in Kerala. Hence religious tolerance and secular attitudes are deeprooted in the heterogenous population of Kerala, which might be on account of the modernization and social change that swept the length and breadth of Kerala, particularly during the recent half century since independence.

During the period of Kerala's isolated growth, caste was the greatest single force of stratification in the society. The caste system which prevailed in Kerala was different from the rest of India. Of the four orthodox 'varnas' of the code of Manu, virtually only the first (the Brahmins) and the last (the Sudras) are represented among the indigenous castes of Kerala. Certain castes in Kerala claim to be and assume the name and occupations of the Kshatriyas or Vaisyas, but were not acknowledged to be in existence in the past within Kerala. When we consider the Hindus, the caste system presents yet another complex characteristic of the people of Kerala. It did not exist in ancient Kerala Society (Aiyappan, 1982). The caste system with its religious and social exclusiveness had not crystallised itself during the early Sangam age and the later Sangam period. It was an innovation introduced by the Aryans, who came here from outside (Menon, 1977). By the eighth century A.D., the Aryanisation of Kerala reached its peak. The Brahmins attained a position of primacy in social and religious matters during the age of the Kulasekharan of Mahodayapuram (A.D. 800 - 1102). The Kshatriyas ruling class and the Nayars (Warriors) who constituted powerful elements of the population had come under the effective grip of the Brahmins. The Ezhavas (Toddy tappers) the Kammalars (Artisans), the Mukkuvars (Fisherfolk) and several other castes, who engaged themselves in occupations which involved manual labour were the main castes that constituted the lower strata in society and they were subjected to gross social disabilities. This system further accentuated the process of stratification of social groups and developed a peculiar structure, the caste system, which required the organization of agrarian life on the feudal model. Today, the major castes of Kerala are: Namboodiris, Kshatriyas, Nayars, Ezhavas, Artisans and Scheduled Castes and Scheduled Tribes.

Namboodiris

The Namboodiris form the highest caste in Kerala. Though numerically small, they held a prominent position in society in the past as they were the high priests as well as the Jenmis. They were the custodians of the Vedas. On the basis of certain rights and privileges they were divided into the following groups: (i) performing holy sacrifices; (ii) teaching the Vedas and Sastras; (iii) officiating as family priests; (iv) becoming sanyasis; (v) officiating priests in temples; (vi) studying the Vedas; (vii) cooking for all classes of Namboodiris; and (viii) taking part in the performance of sastrangam (Menon, 1977).

Nampoothiripad (1952) wrote that the 'Namboodiris probably recruited and made Brahmins, of native men and women from among what he terms "the original Nayars" a casteless, but a slightly stratified matrilineal people, a little more developed than the food-gatherers'. Namboodiris follow the patrilineal family system. Their house is traditionally known as 'Illam'. The patrilineal family organization of the Namboodiri Illam was characterised by two important features - indivisibility of the joint family property and the caste injunctions that only the eldest brother was allowed to marry within the caste and the other males could only follow 'sambandham' or liaison with female of any of the high caste Kshatriyas and Nayars (Rao, 1957).

Namboodiris today are not the same group of population as their traditional ancestors. Today they are economically poor, and mostly living in nuclear families, they do not follow the traditional attitude towards pollution with its old intensity, they take food from hotels and other public places, have inter-caste marriages often with women of other castes and their men have moved to many modern categories of occupations. Their political consciousness and participation in public life are well known; the first communist Chief Minister of the democratically elected communist party in the World was Mr. E.M.S. Namboothiripad, who happened to be an important Brahmin. Today he is the General Secretary of the Marxist Communist Party of India. He does not practise any Brahminical rituals and traditions. Similarly, many other Brahmins have either partially or fully moved away from the traditional form of Brahminical life. Their hypergamous marriage with Nayar women and migration from the rural to the urban areas and other states in India made them secular and modern. Over and above all these, the attainment of modern higher education extensively noticed among the Brahmins in general, transformed them into a fairly modern society. Such developments have also contributed to relatively better health, low mortality and low fertility among them, which require further empirical validation. However, they are negligible in the study area, hence only a few of them formed the respondents of this study.

Kshatriyas

The Kshatriyas who were next in the order of social precedence also formed a smaller section of the population. They were the rulers and owned huge proportions of land. According to historian's view that the highest ranking Kshatriyas are the koil tampuran category to which belong the lineages of Kottayam, Beypore, Cochin and Kodungallur (Aiyappan, 1982). The caste of Kshatriyas known as Tirumulpad, is concentrated mostly in central Kerala. According to the 1891 Madras Census report, there are two sections of Tirumulpads, one Samanta similar to the Eradis, Nedungadis the other Kshatriya sect. Whether Samanta or Kshatriya, they are all matrilineal and their women are married to Namboodiris. The touch of these females does not pollute the Namboodiris and food cooked by them may be eaten by the latter (Ibid.). Today the position is not the same, like Brahmins and Nayars; their lifestyles also have changed. Economically most of them are very rich. They are also one of the most highly educated and modernized groups of people in Kerala. Now most of them hold very high positions in the states as well as in the Central Government. But numerically they are one of the smallest caste groups. However, the present sample does not include the Kshatriyas.

Nayars

The Nayars who were placed next below the Brahmins and Kshatriyas constitute a considerable bulk of the population. The term Nayar originated from the word 'nayakar' which means leader in the fields of administration and war. They formed the most powerful section of the Hindu community in the past but not today. In ancient and medieval times they played the role of 'protector' caste, which bore the responsibility of defending the country and keeping law and order. In the medieval set-up the Nayars had to render political and civil services and it was their duty to safeguard the right of other classes. They were distinguished into high caste and low caste sudras. The sub-divisions of the Nayars are the most bewildering. Many authors have given slightly varying divisions depending upon regional differences. According to Rao (1957), the following may be taken as fairly representing the whole region; (i) Kiriyathil Nayar; (ii) Illathu Nayar; (iii) Swarupathil Nayar; (iv) Idacheri Nayar; (v) Agattucharna and Purattucharna; (vi) Seethikan; (vii) Padamangalam; (viii) Tamil Padakkar; (ix) Maran; (x) Pallichan; (ix) Vattekad (xii) Chembotti and service castes like (a) Vilakkithala Nayar (barber), and (b) Veluthedathu Nayar (Washerman). Some of the high caste Nayars served the Namboothiris as domestic servants (Illakars) and some formed the militia of the country (Swaroopam), (Mencher and Ramanunni, 1979, Menon, 1967). Marriages among these sub-castes were strictly prohibited in the past but now no restrictions exist. The low caste Nayars were mostly oilmongers, washerman and barbers.

The joint family or large 'taravad' was the chief characteristic of the Nayar way of life. The eldest male member of the 'taravad' was the Karanavan (Uncle) and his nephews were termed the 'Anantharavan'. They also maintained the polyandrous type of marriage. The succession in the family was from Karanavan to Anantharavan and not from father to son. The Nayar's followed the matrilineal system of inheritance (Marumakkathayam). According to the matrilineal system of inheritance, property rights rest exclusively with the women. The full impact of 'Marumakkathayam' on women's status has not been studied in detail even today. According to Wood Cock, (1967) "probably the most important effect of matrilineal (Marumakkathayam) system is that it had left Malayali women with an influence and independent outlook, which one will not find anywhere else in India." Under this system, all children born to the female line had equal right of family property, while only male members, not their children, enjoyed this right. The 'taravad' catered to the physical and intellectual development of its members. Each taravad maintained a 'Kalari' (a Centre of learning and military training), where its members - both men and women were trained in physical fitness and in the arts of traditional warfare, and especially in fighting duels. Tara or Kara was the local community association of Nayars.

Nayars today are entirely different from what they were in the past. Their joint family system, landlordship, leadership in the village, matrilineal inheritance, extensive participation in warfare training, polyandrous type of marriages, etc., have almost changed. Their economic deterioration is widely noticed in most families. No doubt, most of them have attained modern education. They also hold several important administrative bureaucratic, ambassadorial and scientific positions all over India and abroad. At one time after independence, the single largest number of ICS and IAS officers holding the positions of secretaries and ambassadors in India and abroad were Nayars. A few notable such representatives were:

V.K. Krishna Menon, K.P.S. Menon, V.P. Menon, Sardar K.M. Panicker, V.R. Pillai, V.K.B. Pillai, M.K. Vellody and many others. Politically also many Nayars have held the position of Chief Ministers and Ministers in the state and at the Centre. Similarly, several notable scientists and social scientists in the state and in the country belong to the Nayar community. This upward occupational mobility made the community modern. Added to these changes, their migration to urban areas, other states in India and to other countries is very extensive, which also made them modern in their life style, attitude, hygienic practices and reduction in morbidity, mortality and fertility. Today, though a large proportion of rural Nayar people are economically not sound, they are educated, modern, politically conscious and well-organised. A powerful Nayar Service Society (NSS) has branches throughout the state which owns hundreds of schools, colleges and hospitals besides several thousands acres of estate land. The NSS grew from strength to strength, thanks to the dynamic leadership of the late Sri Mannat Padmanabha, who is considered even today as the supreme leader of the Nayar community. They were include in the present study on the basis of their extensive availability in the study area.

Ezhavas and Thiyyas

Ezhavas and Thiyyas form numerically the largest section of the Hindu community. The term Ezhava also has a number of explanations put forward by the people of this community, as well as by the scholars, who have studied them. As the word Izham means toddy, and Izhavas in general followed the profession of toddy tapping, it is very likely that the name may be associated with their traditional calling (Aiyappan, 1982). Toddy tapping and cultivation of palm trees was their traditional main occupation. Originally they were labourers and agriculturists and a few are engaged in business. The social inferiority stamped on the Ezhavas naturally shut them out from all fields of education in the past. For years they remained uneducated. After the temple entry proclamation, the conditions of

Ezhavas started changing. Sri Narayana Guru, the social reformer, who belonged to this community played a great role in the emergence of Ezhavas from their utter backwardness. His religious teachings consisting of the doctrine "one caste, one religion and one God", influenced the people and Kerala society in particular. He united and strengthened the community. Now a major proportion of the people are economically comparable or even equal to the Nayars. In every field of life changes have taken place. Politically and socially they became one of the most powerful groups in the state, when the communist government came into power. Like NSS, their organization is called Sri Narayana Dharma Paripalana Yogam (SNDP) which also has many educational, medical and other social institutions all over the state. A major proportion of the men are working of Gulf countries and this helped to improve their economic and social status during the recent past. Though they have advanced in many facets of life, administratively they are categorized as a backward community. In the present sample, respondents from the Ezhava community find due representation in view of their availability in the study area.

Artisans (Kammalars)

Artisans of Kerala are divided into Assari, Moosari, Thattan, Kollan, Kallassary, etc., according to their hereditary occupations. Educationally and economically they were backward class people, but now a days due to the migration to the Gulf countries, they have better avocations which have made them economically better off. Though statistics are not available, at least 50 per cent of their population would have moved to higher occupational categories. They also enjoy the privileges of reservations in the field of education and employment. Under new schemes introduced by the Central and State governments, they have also secure liberal loans and institutional and financial assistance to improve their traditional occupations. Hence, they no longer belong to the poorest among the poor communities in Kerala. Like Ezhavas, they have also been included in this study.

Scheduled Castes

They were considered untouchables in the past. They fall outside the caste hierarchy and were at the lowest level in society. The most common scheduled caste people in South Kerala are: Pulayars, Parayars, Kuravars, Cherumars etc. According to the 1981 census, they constitute 10 per cent of the total population. The socio-economic status of these groups is the lowest among all the communities. Up to the beginning of the 20th century they worked as bonded labourers. The majority of the large scheduled castes continue to be engaged in agricultural labour. Among the agricultural labourer castes a new political awareness has led many to give up some of their traditional practices (Mencher, 1976). Ayyankali, a well know social reformer, who belonged to this community, played an important role in the improvement of these people. Now the government is implementing several measures for the uplift of these communities. Ever since the Communist government came into power on several occasions in Kerala, special programmes were launched to improve the lot of these people. No doubt, other governments also initiated several programmes which also benefited them. Conversion of some of these people to Christianity rapidly made them modern: Though formal and non-formal education, availability of extensive education and economic support given for their education made them literate during a short period of time. Their socio-economic status today is far better off than that of their counterparts in other states in India. No longer are they backward, at least in the field of education. They also constitute a part of the sample population of the Hindus.

Christians

The history of Christianity in Kerala is the history of the rise and growth of different denominations. "If Asia is known as the cradle of the religions of the World", says a writer in the St. Thomas Christian's Encyclopeadia, "Kerala may be described as the nursery of Christian denominations in the World" (Menon, 1979), A.L. Basham has expressed the view that, "At the time contact between India and the west was close and as an enterprising missionary could easily have travelled from Palestine to India". Be that as it may, Christianity seems to have made definite gains in Kerala during the fifteenth century prior to the arrival of the Portuguese (1498). One of the factors which contributed to the Portuguese to proselyte Christianity was the tolerant policy followed by the native Hindu rulers (Ibid). In Kerala, the Latin Catholics who were converted by St. Francis Xavier in the 16th century formed about half the number of the Christians. According to one account, Syrian Christians were the descendants of high caste Hindu converts made by St. Thomas the apostle in the 1st century, A.D. Another legend traces the origin of Kerala Christian back to Thomas of Cana, a merchant from West Asia, who settled in Kerala with his followers and made converts in the 4th century A.D. Conversion from several castes to Christianity became common during the Portuguese, Dutch and British periods of Kerala history (Aiyappan, 1982). According to the 1901 to 1971 censuses, the number of Christians has gone up from 15.4 to 21.05 per cent. The Christians of St. Thomas in Kerala today are divided mainly into five branches, i.e. (i) the Roman Catholic church following three different rites, viz., Syriac, Latin and Malayalam; (ii) the Jacobite or Orthodox Syrian Church; (iii) the Church of the East or the Nestorian Church; (iv) the Marthoma Syrian Church and (v) the Anglican Church, which is part of the Church of South India. In addition, there are a number of minor denominations, such as the Bible Mission, the Pentecost Mission, the Brother Mission, the Salvation Army and so on (Menon, 1979:184). George Kurian (1942) described rural Syrian Christian groups in Kerala as mostly planters and businessmen with a "fairly high standard of living." He further concludes that "Christians have shown significant changes in their attitudes towards marriage and family" (Mencher and Ramanunni, 1979). The respondents of the present study belongs mainly to the Fishermen Christians who are mostly latin Catholic. The Fishermen Christians predominantly inhabit the coastal belt of Kerala. They also belong mostly to the Catholic denomination. They form the late comers in the field of Christianity through recent conversions from the backward Hindus. They continue to follow the traditional occupation of fishing. A negligible proportion of their community, however, became prosperous by turning to mechanised fishing during the recent past. But most of them still continue to be economically and socially backward (Gulati, 1979). Their literacy level is one of the poorest in Kerala, despite the availability of schools all over the state. No doubt, their food intake includes the optimum consumption of protein through fish (Gulati, 1979). Their level of modernisation is much lower compared to the rest of the population in the state, except for the tribals. Morbidity, mortality and fertility are generally higher in this community

Muslims

Islam seems to have been introduced in Kerala by the Arab traders as early as the seventh or the eighth century A.D. Islam advanced in Kerala only by slow stages. In the course of centuries, it made progress and today, next to Hinduism and Christianity, it is the most important religion in the state. The tolerant policy of the native rulers was a potent factor in the progress of this faith (Menon, 1979). The Zamorin of Calicut deliberately encouraged the lower castes to become Muslims in order to have sufficient sailors to man his warships. However, during the time of Portuguese and Dutch, the traditional system was not seriously affected. Changes happened with the invasions of Malabar by Hyder Ali and his son Tippu Sultan. They converted many people to Islam (Mencher, 1976). According to Logan (1951), "Conversion to Muhammedanism has had a marked effect in freeing the slave caste in Malabar from their former brothrons. By conversion a Cheruman (Harijan) obtains a distinct rise in the social scale, and if the consequence bullied or beaten, the influence of the whole Muhammedan community comes to his aid" (Koya, 1983).

Muslims were mostly concentrated in the Malabar, region. Even their population is higher in Malabar. Socially and culturally, Malabar Muslims are far behind their counterparts of the Travancore region. According to the 1971 Census, Muslims constitute 19.5 per cent of the population of Kerala. From 1901 to 1971, their population has gone up from 17.7 to 19.5 per cent. They are by tradition mostly business people. Agriculturists and cultivators are very rare among this community. Now economically most of them are better off due to Gulf influence. But their educational status constitutes to be very low compared to the Hindus and the Christians. The Muslims of Travancore are, however, more educated, better off and modernized than their counterparts in Malabar region. In the present study the Muslims are represented from the Travancore region only.

Dimensions of Social Change

The genesis of rapid social change in Kerala began in the 19th century which witnessed the emergence of a new social order in Kerala under the impact of diverse social, economic and cultural influences.

The British and Indian administrators, who were motivated by liberal impulses, introduced even in the early decades of the 19th century a series of administrative and social reforms with a view to modernizing administration and society in Kerala (Menon, 1979). Rao (1957), in his book on social change in Malabar, has described the Society and Culture of Kerala very broadly as the sum total of all the activities that were grouped under six heads, viz., occupational activities, family life, religious activities, educational activities, leisure time activities and community activities. In the light of these theoretical developments, a resume of social change in Kerala as outlined by Rao and the social history of Kerala by Sreedhara Menon have been taken as a model which has been briefly discussed to highlight the salient aspects of the change in Kerala and Travancore in particular. Since social change cannot be fully documented here without a definite base line study held similarly in the past, only the secondary source of data is considered in this chapter to focus on the general social change in Kerala. However, the dimensions of social change focussed on here relate to those aspects that have very great relevance to fertility behaviour. No doubt, all the dimensions of social change outlined by Rao (Ibid) may be theoretically interesting and demographically relevant but sufficient data is also not available to deal with all of them at length. The salient aspects of social change that are focussed on here relate to: changes in caste structure and its boundaries; education; literary contributions; libraries and mass media; voluntary organizations and movements; land reforms; migration; health delivery system, other governmental efforts and emancipation of women.

Decline of Caste Stratification

The abolition of slavery was one of the important steps taken in Travancore, Cochin and Malabar towards the establishment of a new social order. Kerala was the first state in India to disown the caste system, a reform backed at least by the educated elite, communists and social reformers. The famous Temple Entry Proclamation issued by the Maharaja of Travancore in 1936, opened Hindu temples to people of all castes and creeds. Thus, in Kerala, untouchability was abolished two decades before it was banned in the rest of India (1956). The caste system has broken down in Kerala owing to a variety of causes. Due to the influence of Western education, social reform movements, voluntary organizations like the Nayar Service Society, SNDP, Sahodara Samajam, etc., great changes have been made in the lower classes of society. These organizations were mostly founded for the purpose of eradicating the evils of the caste system. The Vaikom Satyagraha (1924) and the Guruvayoor Satyagraha (1931-32) were important landmarks in the annals of this epic fight for the eradication of untouchability in Kerala (Iyer, 1970). In the wake of the far-reaching changes that have taken place in the functioning of the caste system, the institution of sub-castes has also almost disappeared from Kerala. Inter-community dining between all castes and communities is now the order of the day; not only inter-dining, but also inter-marriage between members of the erstwhile sub-castes has become an accepted social reality today. In this context, it is relevant to examine the levelling up of sub-caste boundaries among the Nayars. Among the Nayars two things happened with respect to social change in the past. On the one hand, the increased mobility and especially the gradual breakup of the large 'taravads', led to a far larger number of Nayar sub-caste being represented in many areas. On the other hand, there has been a movement towards breaking down of Nayar sub-caste distinctions and an attempt to unite all Nayars. This breakdown of Nayar sub-caste distinctions has occurred more in Travancore than elsewhere. Mencher in 1959 wrote that many of the younger Nayars today did not even know to what sub-caste they belong (Mencher and Ramanunni, 1976).

Caste and Politics

The caste system in Kerala has changed beyond recognition, though it has not lost its grip on the public mind. Very few people would dare defend caste openly today. The people of each caste prefers to educate their children in schools and colleges run by them and the various castes in Kerala have established their own educational institutions. These remain centres of communalism and caste. Caste considerations do influence voting in elections (Puthenkalam, 1977). Mencher (1976), in her essay on anthropological research in Kerala, referred to the present situation of caste in the following lines: "It is true that inter-caste barriers in Kerala have broken down and caste consciousness is less pronounced in the minds of the people of the present generation, but it is doubtful whether the caste system can be said to have died out completely. A keen observer of the social scene in Kerala cannot fail to note the fact that caste has entered another arena, viz., that of modern politics, and that many of the inequalities of the caste system are still operative to Kerala". There was always a correlation between caste and politics (Mencher, 1976).

Education and Change

Education broke up the old concept of society and introduced new factors of social change. The social changes in the wake of English education affected every sphere of life. The English and Vernacular schools replaced traditional education and the Namboodiris' monopoly. The British Administration recognized no caste barriers in the matter of recruitment to the services, though this was not fully true of the administration of Travancore and Cochin, where people belonging to upper castes were patronised by the princely order. However, the democratisation of education began only at the start of the nineteenth century, when the state not only undertook the opening of schools on a large scale, but made them available to children of all castes and creeds. Women, Muslims and the untouchables received special encouragement in these schools (Nayar, 1986). According to the census of 1901, Travancore was foremost among the Indian states in both general education and women's education. Lord Curzon, Viceroy and Governor-General of India, visited Travancore in the first decade of the twentieth century and the sight that pleased him most was the vast array of bright-eyed students, girls, who were called upon together to receive him (Aiyar, 1923). The development of education in the state owes much to the importance given to it in the Kerala culture and to the work done by the European Missionaries. The rulers of both Travancore and Cochin gave considerable impetus to education by having the state pay the entire cost of primary education. These official efforts were supplemented by private efforts which began with the establishment of Church-managed schools and colleges, by foreign Christian missionaries. The first Christian college was established at Kottayam in 1813. The formal channels of education, i.e., the schools and colleges managed by the government, by private persons, or by other organizations, are recognized by the appropriate government agencies (Kerala State Education Department and University). The ideology embodied in the modern educational system is to breed a scientific spirit (Puthenkalam, 1977). The structure of the educational system radically differs from the old type by adapting itself to changing ideas. The school life of the students has grown attractive with the growth of extra-curricular activities. The work of the Christian missionaries and the spread of western education helped to bring about a radical social change. Kerala had 12,120 schools and 168 colleges by 1985 (D.P.I. 1985). Most of them are run by private agencies. Out of the total number of colleges, 132 are run by voluntary agencies and only 36 are in the public sector. These voluntary efforts of different communities have assisted people through formal and informal education, developed their health facilities and offered scope for further advancement in life, which would have contributed directly to fertility decline. Nevertheless, education has spread differentially among the three religious groups; it is near universal among the Hindus, but not so among the other two communities.

Literary Contributions

The nature of the evolution of literature from religious to secular themes is also a great factor of social change. The change in the attitude and contact of literature came about only by the end of the nineteenth century. Novels made their appearance about this time. Social themes were dealt with even in the very first novels like 'Kundalatha', 'Indulekha' and 'Sarada'. In the drama also, the modern trend is towards the portrayal of real life. The realistic plays of writers like Thoppil Bhasi, K.T. Mohammad, Ponkunnam Varkey and M.P. Chellappan Nayar dealt with stark poverty and social injustice. Thoppil Bhasi, through his series of revolutionary dramas, frequently performed all over the state, influenced people against several outdated customs like ostracism of leprosy patients and promoted a secular value system and socialism. He is largely instrumental in spreading communism fast in Kerala through his novel,"You Made me a Communist" (Ningal Enne Communistaki). Some of the great novels of modern writers like Thakazhi, and Kesavadeve have been filmed and their message was spread to larger audiences in this way. Modern literacy critics like Joseph Mundassery and the late M.P. Paul have emphasized the point that literature is to be evaluated not only in terms of literature but in terms of life itself. Modern Malayalam poets like Kumaran Assan, Vallathol, Vayalar Ramavarma, etc., and their works also affected to a great extent the momentum of continuing social change throughout Kerala.

Libraries and Mass Media

The library movement in Kerala had its origin in the early part of the nineteenth century. Libraries came into being as a result of the interest taken by the Government as well by the public. The public library at Trivandrum was established in 1829, which is one of the oldest of its kind in India. The successful functioning of the Trivandrum public library came as an eye opener to people within and outside the state. Subsequently, several public libraries were get use in important centres. The Government of Cochin took an active interest in the growth of libraries and this contributed substantially to the progress of the library movement in the area. At present 4,977 (1985) libraries are functioning all over the State and most of them are run on a cooperative basis by the people themselves. Meanwhile, the Government and municipalities in the State take an interest in the library movement. There are recognized and grant-receiving libraries, but there are many non-recognized libraries which exist in the villages. It is, unique feature in the world. In addition to these libraries, Kerala Grandhasala Sangham (Library Co-operative) had thousands of libraries under its patronage.

Newspapers and Periodicals

In Kerala, newspapers and periodicals act as a catalytic agent for social change. Numerous newspapers and magazines are published. The history of journalism in Malayalam commences with the publication of the Rajyasamacharam (News of the country) from Illikunnu in Tellicherry in June, 1847. The credit for bringing out this pioneering publication goes to the German missionary, Dr. Gundert (Menon, 1979). The progress of Malayalam journalism since the turn of the century has been rapid. The most important Malayalam dailies published in Kerala are: *Malayala Manorama, Mathrabhumi, Kerala Kaumudy, Desabhimani and Janayugam.* These dailies had a circulation of more than five lakhs within the country and abroad. In addition, a number of magazines, weeklies, periodicals, etc., are published in various places in Kerala. One of the Malayalam weeklies viz., 'Mangalam', has the highest circulation of any weekly all over the country.

Radio and Television

Radio and television are the important media of cultural expression. The radio broadcast service in Kerala was started as early as March 12, 1943 at Trivandrum. Now All-India Radio has opened stations at Calicut, Trichur and Alleppey to serve people in all parts of the state more effectively. In addition to radio, television also opened a station at Trivandrum recently. The cultural and social programmes broadcasted through these media helped a lot to improve the life-style of the people.

Voluntary Organization's Movements

Voluntary efforts have proved to be equally important and have contributed to allround social development. Various voluntary organizations occupy a prominent place in the social structure. These are voluntary associations on the basis of religion, caste, political parties, employment, art, literature, etc.

By the early decades of the 20th century, all the religious communities in Kerala were affected by powerful reform movements led by such organizations as the Ramakrishna Mission, the Theosophical Society and the Arya Samaj which helped to create in the minds of the Hindus of Kerala a keen awareness of the evils of the caste system. The Hindu reform movements were led by two outstanding leaders of non-Brahmin communities, viz., Sri Chattampi Swamikal, a Nayar Sanyasi and Sri Narayana Guru an Ezhava saint.

Hindu Reforms : Sreedhara Menon in his book on Social and Cultural History of Kerala described the contributions made by these social reformers. For example, Chattampi Swamikal who was born in a Nayar family. During his younger days he actively participated in the war against social and religious evils of the society. The religious and philosophical discourses of Chattampi Swamikal won for him a wide circle of disciples. He acted and spoke strongly against Brahmin domination. His main achievement as a social religious reformer was that he aroused the social consciousness of the members of his own caste, viz., the Nayars and made them fight against the evils that had crept into their ranks. The work of Chattampi Swamikal considerably helped the Nayar Service Society and its leaders viz., Mannath Padmanabhan, in their efforts to bring about the moral regeneration of the community by eradicating such social evils of untouchability and sub-caste barriers, stop social practices like Talikettu Kalyanam, Tirandukuli, etc., which had impoverished many a middle-class Nayar family. He also infused new life and vigour into Hinduism at a time when it was facing threat of conversions from within its fold to Christianity and Islam.

Like Chattampi Swamikal, Sri Narayana Guru also revolted against the existing social order in which the Brahmins enjoyed a position of primacy. He was born in a middle-class Ezhava community. He was closely associated with the Sri Narayana Dharma Paripalana Yogam (SNDP), the representative organization of the Ezhavas. He gave the Hindu religious movement a social content and a practical turn in Kerala. Sri Narayana Guru set up shrines dedicated to 'Siva' as a parallel system to that of the caste Hindus, who denied the entry of the Ezhavas in their temples. The religious revival initiated by Sri Narayana Guru contributed a great deal to the promulgation of the famous Temple Entry Proclamation of November, 1936. He also fought against irrational practices such as Talikettu Kalyanam, Tirandukuly, Pulikudi etc., which stood in the way of progress. He preached against the evil of drink and enunciated the famous doctrine "One caste, one religion, one God for man". Another famous saying of Sri Narayana Guru was, "Whatever be one's religion, it is enough if the individual become good. He also advocated inter-marriages between different castes as a means of achieving social cohesion and evolving a classless and casteless society. His teachings have contributed a great deal in transforming the backward classes on modern lines.

As a follower of Chattampi Swamikal, Mannath Padmanabhan carried forward the message of modernization till the recent past. He institutionalised Nayar society, eradicated outdated rituals, customs and extravagant expenditure among the Nayars. His pioneering efforts in establishing many schools and colleges rapidly and extensively improved the educational standards of the Nayars and other communities. His effort also enabled them to accelerate pace of occupational mobility among the Nayars. The Nayars emerged as a political force with considerable power during his time. Their influence has declined after independence, though they were powerful leaders earlier. Today the NSS is one of the largest voluntary organization in Kerala and India.

In addition to Chattampi Swamikal and Sri Narayana Guru, another major social and religious leader was Ayyankali, a popular leader who founded the Sadhu Jana Paripalana Yogam. Other leaders who either directly or indirectly drew inspiration from Sri Narayana Guru were Dr. Palpu, Kumaran Assan, Ayyappan, R. Sankar, Nataraja Guru and Nityachaithanyayati. Those who were similarly influenced by the teachings of Chattampi Swamikal include Sri Nilakanta Tirthapada Swamikal, who played a leading role in all reform movements, particularly in the campaign against untouchability and eradication of many other social evils. In addition to the reform movements led by Chattampi Swamikal and Sri Narayana Guru, the All India religious and social reform movements like the Arya Samaj, Ramakrishna Mission and Theosophical Society had their marginal influence on certain sections of Hindu society. Among all these, Ramakrishna Mission had a great influence. Swami Vivekananda played an important role in the activities of this society.

Movements for Christian Unity: The religious movements within the Christian Churches in Kerala derived not only to unite the different sections of the Christian community owing allegiance to different denominations but also to inclined the Church. They believed that for maintaining a proper missionary spirit, it was necessary to integrate the Church effectively in the cultural settings of independent India. However, this aim of the Christians is not yet fully realised even today.

Muslim Reform Movements: The Muslim community of Kerala has also been influenced by the 'wind of change' in recent times. This community produced in recent times some outstanding social and religious leaders who worked hard for its social uplift and moral regeneration (Menon, 1979). Vakkom Abdul Khadar Moulvi, a scholar in Arabic, Persian, Urdu and Malayalam was the pioneer among them. The Muslim Educational Society, which was started in 1964, has taken up the care of Muslim women. It has set up women's sections in many schools both at state and district levels. Though education of girls has received great impetus in Kerala, compared to women in other states, more than 50 per cent of Muslim girls are still illiterate or ignorant in Kerala. The main objective of this society is to educate Muslim women for the social, economic and other development of women. The existing social backwardness of the Muslims in Kerala is largely because of the poor educational attainment of women consequently there is less social change among them compared to other communities.

Land Reforms : One of the most significant developments in the recent political economy of the state is the shift in political power from the rich to the poor. Along with this shift, and as a consequence of it, there has been a considerable transfer of wealth and income to the lower strata of society. These changes have been brought about through land reform, job security, enforcement of minimum wages, pension benefits for agricultural labourers, reservation of places in educational institutions and on public bodies for the economically and socially backward groups in the community (Zachariah, 1983) according to the present Land Reform Act (1957), in Kerala which is, perhaps, the most drastic of any passed by any state legislature in India. It not only provides for an exceptionally low land ceiling but also gives the actual right of ownership of land to the real tiller of the soil. The present act has for the most part benefited the lower middle classes who held land on various kinds of tenure from higher caste landlords or tenants (Mencher, 1976). The Land Reforms Act was finally passed in 1963 and by 1969, tenancy was altogether abolished. Rental income from land was also virtually abolished throughout Kerala. The 1969 amendments to the land reforms act lowered the ceiling to ten acres, removed some of the exemptions from the ceiling, and gave the "hutment dwellers" the right to purchase about one tenth of an acre of land per house-hold at a nominal price. According to Ratcliffe (1978), fertility decline was caused by an increase in the income of the poor resulting from the redistributive policies of the government. One such element is the economic deprivation resulting from the land reforms". Thus, the series of land reforms introduced in Kerala since the latter half of the 19th century have helped in accelerating the pace of social and economic change in the state.

Migration and Social Change

Migration of people, particularly women, makes people rapidly modern, leading to several sequential social changes in a society. It provides non-formal education through direct and indirect means, and exposes people to new and diverse situations it also provides an opportunity to modify and change the traditional life style, customs, habits and behaviour in general. In this context, the people of Kerala are more migratory than their counterparts in other states in India.

They not only migrate to urban areas within Kerala and outside Kerala, but also to countries in West Asia, Europe, America and Asia. According to Nayar's recent study (1983) 60 per cent of the total emigrant workers from Kerala are workers in countrics outside India. It started on a large scale during the last fifty years and reached a peak period during the oil boom in West Asian Countries. Nayar (1983: 9) wrote "Emigration from India to the Gulf countries takes place mainly from seven states - Kerala, Andhra Pradesh, Punjab, Gujarat, Goa, Maharashtra and Tamil Nadu. Of these seven states, Kerala is supposed to account for not less 50 per cent of the migrants. The bulk of the migrants from Bombay (in the state of Maharashtra) are persons belonging to Kerala and Goa. According to a survey conducted in Kerala during January-March, 1980, there were 207.8 thousand persons who had gone abroad for work of whom 186.5 thousands (90%) were in countries in West Asia". Since the vast majority of the migrants are rural people, migration makes them modern in many ways. Their remittance of money to their dependents back home also makes them prosperous in all aspects of life. According to Nayar (Ibid) even the most unskilled and the most low paid workers reportedly remit about Rs. 1,000 per month. Their children get a good education, better nutritional status and all modern amenities of life, which makes the whole family prosperous and modern.

The large scale migration of people from Kerala takes place mainly from the Districts of Trivandrum, Alleppey, Quilon, Kottayam, Ernakulam, Trichur and Malapuram. Except the Malapuram district, which is a predominantly Muslim area, in all other districts, the fertility of the migrants is likely to be lower. In the recent studies carried out in Kerala by Mahadevan (1986, 1987), the migrants demonstrate significantly lower fertility than the non-migrants. Another interesting feature noticed by Nayar is that 35 per cent of the migrants are bachelors below the age of 25, which again reduces their fertility. Hence emigration of people leads to social change, economic prosperity and demographic change. However, in the present study, it is not an objective and hence not considered.

Health Delivery System

The native rulers of Travancore and Cochin took an active part in encouraging public health programmes even in the nineteenth century. They enforced sanitary measures in temples, bazaars and other public places and developed a paramedical public health and sanitation infrastructure in the second half of the nineteenth century. A free hospital was opened in Trivandrum by the Maharaja of Travancore in 1865. The growth in medical facilities in Kerala during the five year period 1973-1977 was several times more than the all-India increase. This is specially true of hospitals, where the growth rate in Kerala was fifteen times more than the all-India growth rate (Nayar, 1986). However, the hospitals in Kerala are evenly distributed throughout the state. Statistics available for 1980 indicate that the average service area of a primary health centre was 232 square kilometers in Kerala as against 563 square kilometers in India. In the case of sub-centres it was 21 square kilometeres in Kerala and 63 square kilometers in India. The number of hospital beds per lakh population in the 1984-1985 period was 125 in Kerala and 70 in India. The proportion of doctor-population ratio also showed marked difference. In Kerala, it was 46 per lakh population in 1981, but in India only 39 (Directorate of Health Services, 1985). A recent study in Neyyatinkara Taluk of Trivandrum district revealed that over 75 per cent of the people make use of the services of the primary health centre as against less than ten per cent services of a comparable Pulicherla primary health centre in Chittoor district of Andhra Pradesh (Mahadevan & Sumangala, 1987).

The state government's expenditure on health was Rs. 14,604/- lakhs (i.e., 14.15% of the total budget) in the 1985-86 period. However, the family planning drive in Kerala gathered momentum only in the second half of the 1960's; the progress achieved thereafter has been creditable. In 1961-62, the percentage of eligible couples protected was 0.82, but in 1982-83, it was 33.5 per cent; during the same period, the all-India average was 25.9 per cent (Family Welfare, 1982-83).

The physical environment in most parts of Kerala is healthy and that is a major factor for the low mortality and fertility in Kerala. Kerala also has a long native tradition of medical treatment (Ayurvedic System). The rulers of the state have always taken great interest in health matters and have committed sufficient public funds for both curative and preventive medicine. In addition, the foreign missionaries established private hospitals and trained health personnel in large numbers (Zachariah, 1983). Personal hygiene is also an important factor for the better health of Keralites. Some foreign writers have drawn special attention to these aspects. The Malayali, irrespective of caste or community, gets up early in the morning and attends to his morning routine of cleaning teeth and tongue, having a daily oil bath, etc. These habits are a must for the Malayali (Menon, 1979). Another important factor that positively influences better health in Kerala is the good transport facilities that provide the access to medical facilities. Good communication enables newspaper to reach every corner of the state. Also, the high literacy rate in Kerala helped in the quick delivery of the government's health care and family planning inputs. Thus, health conditions, in Kerala have always been better than those in other parts of India and the low fertility, mortality and high performance of family planning in Kerala also been on account of the extensive coverage of public health services by a comprehensive health care system by government and voluntary agencies alike.

Other Developmental Programmes

Rural development forms the key for increasing the purchasing power of people and their capacity to accept modern innovations in all walks of life. The development of rural areas makes any region or country really progressive. The wide disparity between villages and cities that exists in other states of India is not seen in Kerala. Rural development programmes were started all over the state as early as 1950s. During the First and Second Plan periods, community development work was in full swing ever since the blocks were created. Through the rural development agencies, houses for poor people have been built in most villages, and house sites have been distributed to others. Through the minimum needs programmes, loans for self-employment, animal and agricultural inputs have been made available to people. For the care of pre-school children and pregnant mothers, numerous Anganwadi centres came into being in most places in the state and they have contributed extensively to the health of poor mothers and children. In addition to this, thanks to the higher level of education and widespread transport facilities, utilization of the existing developmental inputs has dramatically risen in Kerala which is not the case in many other states in India.

Emancipation of Women

Emancipation is an outstanding characteristic of the women of

Kerala, which distinguishes them from their counterparts elsewhere in India. This is not only reflected in education and occupation, but also in their higher age at marriage, higher acceptance of family planning, active participation in voluntary organizations, politics, etc., (Nayar, 1984). The high status of women in Kerala has a long historical past. It is also influenced by various ecological and sociological factors. Historically the Sangham age was the turning point for women in society. Throughout the Sangham age women enjoyed a high status. They were trained not only in the rituals but in music and dancing. However, the coming of the Aryans to Kerala in large numbers in the subsequent centuries (8th century and later) altered the situation. During that period, the status of Brahmin women in society became worse. The Brahmins introduced the system of child marriage, prohibition of widow remarriage and a host of other practices. At the same time position of Nayar women in society was very prominent. The important reason for the high status of Nayar women was "Marumakkathayam" (Matriliny), the law of inheritance through the female line. It was not only confined to the Nayar community alone, but also to the Kshatriyas, some of the Muslims of Malabar, and many backward communities such as Ezhavas, artisans and tribals like Kurichiyas (Mahadevan, 1979).

Another major index in the status enjoyed by women in Kerala during the same period and modern times was the level, of education attained by them. The 'Palli' was the educational institution; education was offered in Sanskrit and the vernacular for both boys and girls up to 10 years of age. Direct activity of the state in the field of education began only in 1917, when Rani Gouri Parvathi Bhai, the then ruler of Travancore, with the assistance of Devan Munro, introduced free and compulsory education in Travancore for all children (Nayar, Ibid). However, the popularisation of women's education in the 19th century was largely the work of missionaries who opened schools for girls in different parts of Kerala. The rate of growth of female education is still continuing. This state can boast of the highest rate of female literacy in India, which according to the 1981 census was 64.4 per cent. Thus, the number of girls in schools during 1982-83 was 27.4 lakhs, while the number of women who passed S.S.L.C. in 1983 was 38.1 as against 36.4% of boys. There were more than a lakh of women during the same year studying in colleges and Universities. The drop-out rate among girls in the different standards in the schools is the lowest in Kerala as compared to the other states of India (Nair, 1981).

As regards occupational status in traditional Kerala society, by the large, only women in the lower strata went for employment and this was mostly in agriculture but the situation has changed during the last fifty years. The percentage of work participation rates of women in Kerala and in India has decreased over the decades. From 1961 to 1981 it was 19.71 to 17.02 in Kerala and 27.93 to 20.85 in India (Census, 1981). Out of the total number of workers, 43 per cent are agricultural labourers; 44 per cent were working in the service sector and other productive activities. Participation of women in the factory sector is the highest in Kerala compared to the other states in India. There are also a large number of women in the service sector as clerks in banks and offices. Many work as teachers, nurses and a few as professionals and technical personnel (Census, 1981). The percentage of females who are literates but unemployed is also as high as 84 per cent in Kerala. In addition to this, the average age at marriage of women in this part has gone up to 22 years while for India it has only increased to 18 years (Census, 1981). Late marriage enabled women to have better choice of husbands, better understanding of family responsibilities, family planning and child care. This has been a key factor in the steep fertility decline in Kerala in recent years (Nayar, 1981). Hence, 'one is likely to find a sizeable proportion of the female population who are literate but who are neither married nor employed' (Umadevi, 1984).

Another area where women have been able to make an impact on society, in Kerala is in social welfare activities. A study conducted by the Sociology Department of Kerala University (Nayar, 1975) showed that the largest number of voluntary social service agencies existing in Kerala were run by women. Now the growth of Mahilasamajam, Anganwadi, balavadies etc., all over Kerala is tremendous. There were 2,987 Balavadies and 9,493 Mahila Mandals functioning at Block levels (Department of Economics and Statistics, 1982). This partly explains the better status of women for the population as a whole, except, perhaps, among the Muslims, it is one of the major social change, that have taken place in Kerala. Enhancement of status of women naturally would have contributed to the decline in fertility and mortality, which is studied here by considering the age at marriage of women and the opportunity cost perceived by them.

The preceding chapter discusses various dimensions of socia

change, which individually and together, would have contributed to dramatic changes among the population of Kerala by transforming them into a modern society in the short period since the beginning of the 20th century and particularly after independence. Such changes in a developed country of the West would have taken centuries to attain the same level of progress. But such sweeping social changes have not taken place in any other state in India. Even in Kerala, different levels of social change have taken place among the Hindus, Christians and the Muslims. While the Hindus in general, and forward caste Hindus in particular, have attained a higher level of social advancement, similar developments have taken place only among the Christians. The rest of the population is relatively backward in many aspects of life, but even they are much more advanced compared to their counterparts in the rest of India. Therefore, in the field of social change, Kerala presents a unique experience consequent to the progress achieved on specific dimensions of social change. Similarly, the fertility of the different religious groups also differs significantly.

Religion and Differential Fertility

Religion has always been an unique and important facet of human life, it is an intrinsic aspect of the culture of all societies. In a society, religious institutions and their values have specific influence upon fertility. The ancestors and gods of primitive society are its peculiar heritage, and the society has a role of responsibility for the preservation and perpetuation of this heritage (Paul and Paul, 1954). However, fertility differences by religions and ethnic groups are widespread. Religion and ethnicity are associated with differences in norm relating to contraception and abortion and also with different patterns of fertility (Day, 1984). The religious differences in fertility behaviour was first identified through the 'Indianapolis' Study conducted in USA. It revealed that the Catholics have the highest fertility, followed by the Protestants and Jews (Kiser, et al., 1958). On the other hand, Kirck has conclusively confirmed that the muslims in general have very high fertility. In India, from the numerical point of view Hinduism is the major religion followed by islam and Christianity. According to the 1971 census, the Hindus constitute 82.7 per cent of the total population, while for Muslims and Christians, these percentages are 11.2 and 2.0 respectively (Census, 1971).

A number of studies conducted in different parts of India have brought out the religious differences in fertility behaviour between the two major religious groups, viz., the Hindus and Muslims. The Mysore Population Study (U.N., 1961) indicated that religion is associated with fertility; married muslim women have an average of larger number of children than hindus. In central India, Driver (1963) found that the average number of children born to the Hindu and Muslim wives was 4.5 and 4.6 respectively. A study conducted by Kurup and George (1965) in Travancore - Cochin state revealed that the average number of children born to wives who had completed their fertility was 6.4 for the Hindus and 7 for Muslims. Another recent study conducted in Kerala (Zachariah, 1983) found that the average parity of the Muslim women was 4.1, while that of Nayars was only 2.9, a difference of 1.2 children per women. The completed fertility of these two groups differs by 2.5 children. Between Nayars and Latin Christians, the difference in completed fertility was 2.7 children. In the light of the preceding findings it is confirmed that in India the Hindus have the lowest fertility, compared to the Christians and Muslims.

The significant fertility variations which are observed among the three religious groups can be seen in the following table 1.1

Table 1.1: Mean live births, maximum expected and additional family size norms according to the three religious groups

Religious groups	Hindus	Christians	Muslims	Total
Mean live births	2.6	3.5	3.4	2.9
Maximum number of children desired	2.5	3.3	3.1	2.7
Additional children desired	0.5	1.2	1.0	0.7

It is confirmed that fertility is significantly lower among the Hindus. But the difference between the Christians and Muslims is not statistically significant. The other two variables of fertility behaviour, viz., maximum expected number of children and additional expected number of children showed differences in fertility among the three religious groups. It is interesting to note that all the three religious

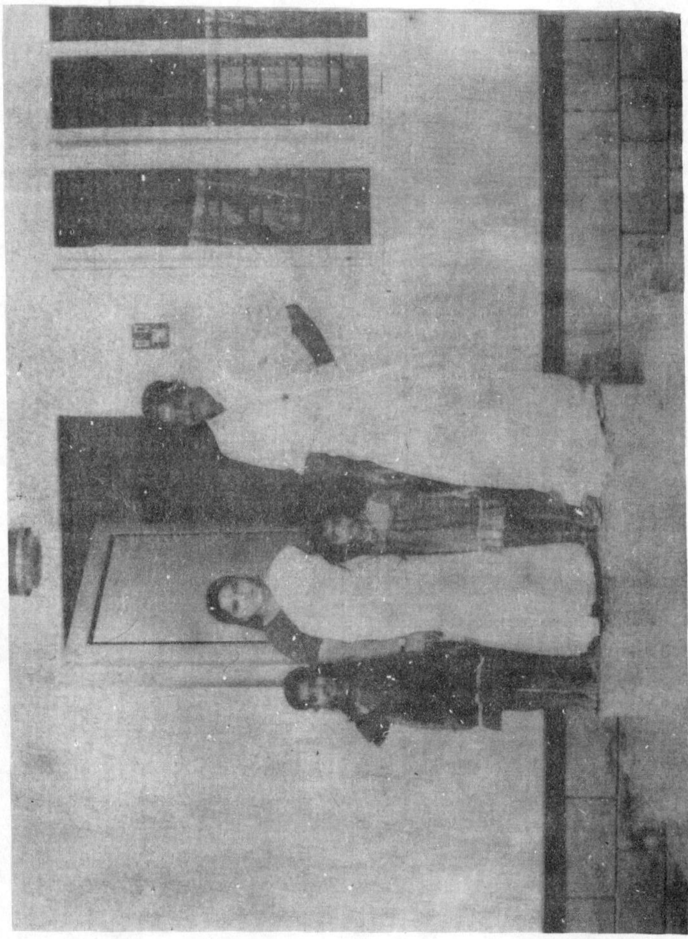

A HINDU (NAIR) FAMILY

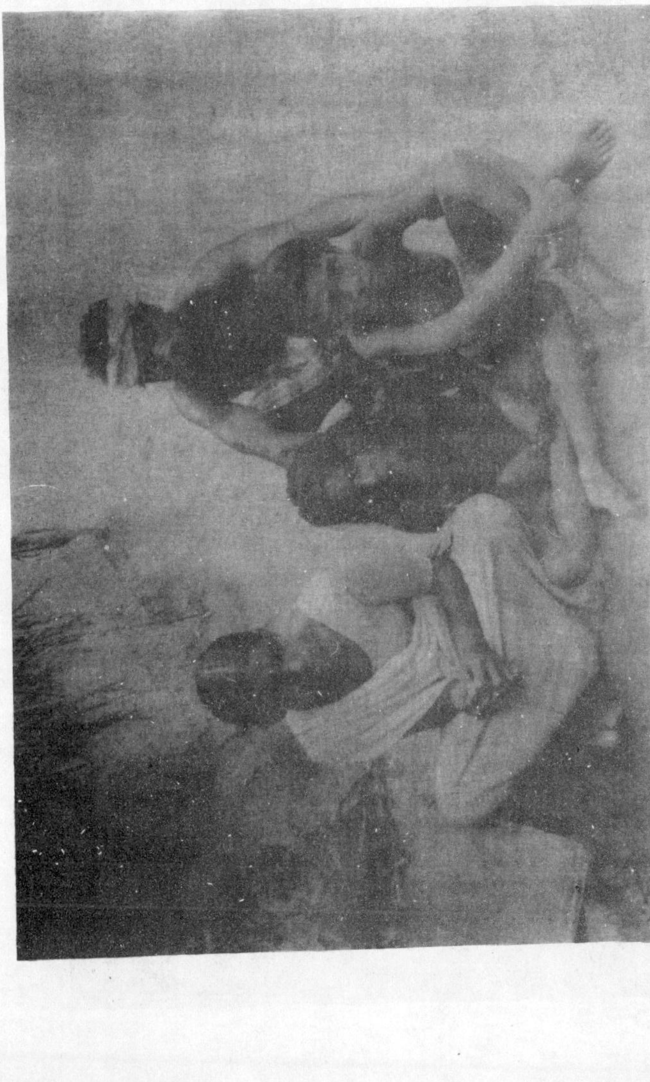

A HINDU (HARIJAN) FAMILY

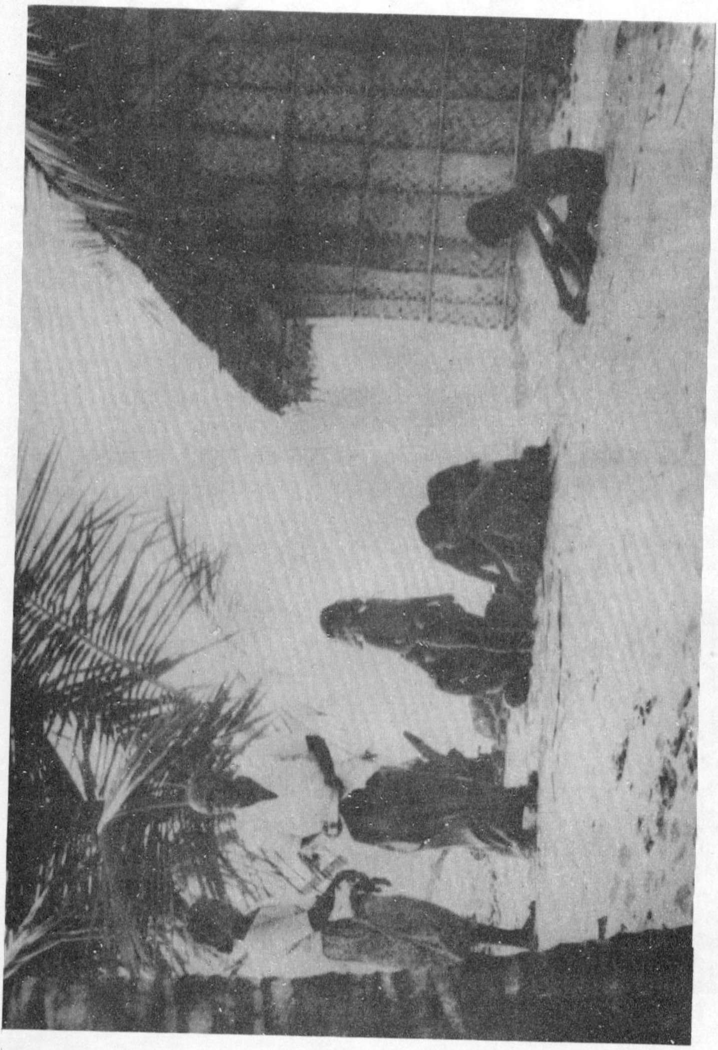

A FISHERMAN CHRISTIAN FAMILY

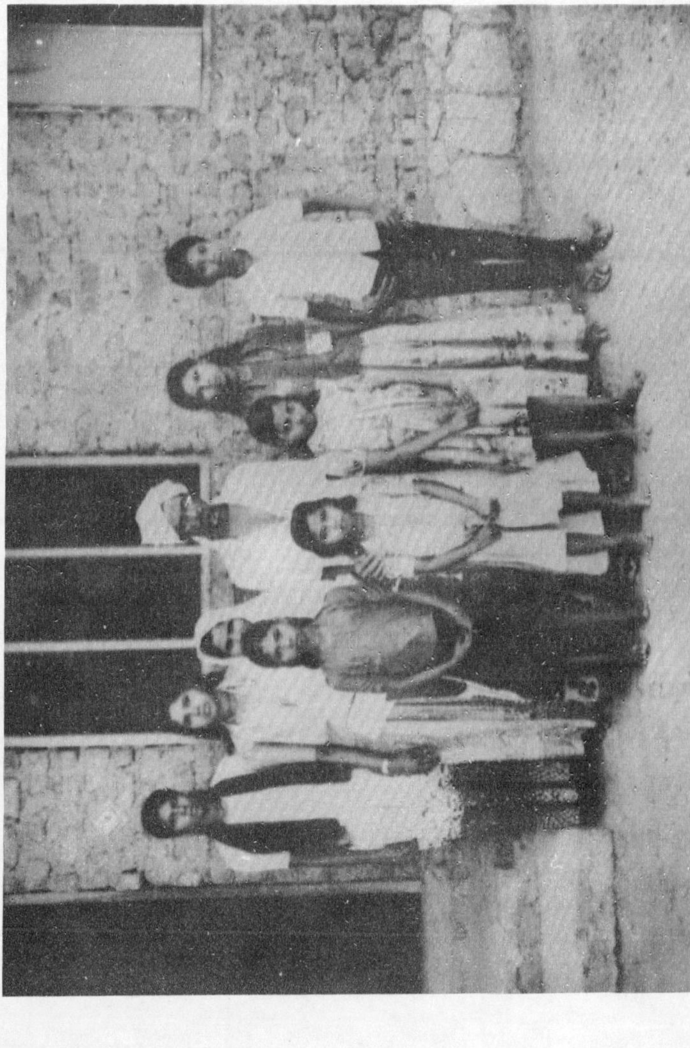

A MUSLIM FAMILY

groups desired slightly less number of children during their life time than what they have already got. As expected, the high fertility groups of Christians and Muslims would like to have 0.2 and 0.3 children respectively and for the Hindus 0.1 less children than their current live births when they stop their family formation. However, the young mothers of these communities prefer again significantly more children among the Christians (1.2) and Muslims (1.0) than among the Hindus (0.5). But, for the population as a whole, the mean live births constitute 2.4, maximum expected children 2.7 and additional expected child 0.7 only. Thus, significant fertility difference is noticed in the light of the present fertility and also in the near future for the Hindus on the one side and Christians and Muslims on the other. Added to these differences of fertility, still higher differences are noticed not only between the Hindus and non-Hindus but also between the Christians and Muslims, when their duration of married life is controlled. In the light of this differential fertility noticed among the Hindus, Christians and Muslims, in the past and also in the present study, an attempt is made here to identify their determinants. The differential social changes which would have contributed to a great extent we have already discussed to fertility differences, the present effort is to go into more specific issues, particularly the influence of intermediate variables, socio-economic status and value of children.

TWO

NUPTIALITY AND FERTILITY

As a social institution universality of marriage was recognized in the history of nuptiality of India. Demographers have long ago recognized marriage as one of the principal proximate determinants of fertility. Malthus (1798) in his thesis on population stated that delay in marriage is a major preventive check of moral restraint on the growth of population. Age at first marriage identifies the onset of exposure to the risk of socially sanctioned child bearing, and, as such, it is a principal determinant of the number of births a woman will have (Bongaarts, 1983).

Age at marriage, a strong point in the reproductive process, is traditionally low in many developing countries as compared to developed countries. Many studies have shown the strong negative relationship between age at marriage and fertility (Mahadevan, 1986 & 1979; Audinarayana, 1985; Zachariah, 1983; Bongaarts, 1983; Wyon & Gordon, 1971; Malini Karkal, 1968; Agarwala, 1965; Freedman, 1963). World Fertility Survey (WFS) has reported "Although age at marriage is a topic of interest to demographers in its own right, it has been singled out for intensive study primarily because of the impact of nuptiality on fertility." In the developed world as a whole, age at marriage is highest and fertility is lowest, but the picture is not the same in the developing countries. Age at marriage has risen in East Asia and in a few countries of South-East Asia, and this might have contributed to the overall decline in birth rates in these countries. However, Indonesia and countries belonging to the Indian subcontinent still have lower ages at marriage, and this provides a partial explanation of high birth rates in those nations (Population Programme News, 1985).

In Kerala where literacy level has increased as high as 70 per cent (1981 Census) the mean age at marriage has also correspondingly increased. According to the 1981 census the mean age at marriage for women was 21.9 and for men 27.2. Education and emancipation of women were the two major factors that strongly influenced the higher age at marriage in Kerala (Zachariah, 1983).

According to the present data, for the population in general the mean age at marriage for females averaged 19.8 years and for males it was 26.2 years. At the same time the mean age at marriage varies according to the religious groups. For women it was highest among the Hindus (20.0) followed by Christians (18.4) and Muslims (17.9). In the case of males also the Hindus have the highest mean age at marriage of 27.1, followed by Muslims 25.4 and the lowest is found among the fishermen Christians (24.5). These variations in age at marriage of boys and girls across these cultural groups might be contributing to their existing variation in fertility which is examined in the table 2.1.

Table 2.1: Percentage distribution of age at marriage of wife by the three religious groups

Age at marriage	Hindus	Christians	Muslims	Total
≤ 12 years	0.2	-	0.7	0.2 (2)
13 - 15	6.7	7.7	13.3	7.9 (79)
16 - 18	27.7	51.1	51.7	36.8 (368)
19 - 21	37.0	30.3	25.8	33.8 (338)
22 - 24	18.7	9.2	8.5	14.9 (149)
25 +	9.7	1.7		6.4 (64)
Total	100.0 (616)	100.0 (233)	100.0 (151)	100.0 (1000)

When data on age at marriage of the wives in general is grouped (see table 2.1) the highest proportion (36.8%) of them got married between the ages of 16 to 18 years. Among the various religious groups the same trend is noticed for the Muslims (51.7%) and Christians (51.1%), but among Hindus the highest percentage (37%) of women got married between the age group of 19-21. The second largest percentage (33.8%) of wives got married in between the age group of 19-21, followed by 15 per cent who married between 22-24. Those who had married at 15 years was only 8 per cent of the total population and the highest age at marriage, i.e., above 25 years of age, constituted only 6.4 per cent. Among the various religious groups the 9.7 per cent of the Hindu girls performed their marriage at the age of 25 years and above and only a negligible percentage of Christians falls under the similar category but Muslims are nil in this group.

Table 2.2 : Percentage distribution of age at marriage of husband by the three religious groups

Age at marriage	Hindus	Christians	Muslims	Total
≤ 19 year	0.8	3.9	0.7	1.5 (15)
20 - 24	26.8	51.9	44.2	35.3 (353)
25 - 29	48.2	36.1	43.7	44.7 (447)
30 - 34	18.5	6.4	8.6	14.2 (142)
35 +	5.7	1.7	2.7	4.3 (43)
Total	100.0 (616)	100.0 (233)	100.0 (151)	100.0 (1000)

In the case of husbands (Table 2.2) 44.7 per cent of marriages took place at the age of 25-29 years, followed by 35.3 per cent between 20-24 years. 14.2 per cent of them got married between 30-34 years of age. Those who were married above 35 years were only 4.3 per cent in the population as a whole and early marriage (at ≤ 19 years) was negligible (1.5%). Among the religious groups, the highest per cent (48.2) of the Hindus got married at the age of 25-29 years, but the highest per cent of Fishermen Christians (51.9%) and Muslims (44.4%) got married at 20-24 years. In the case of early marriage groups i.e., ≤ 19 years the Christians constitute only 3.9 per cent and only a negligible per cent of the Hindus (0.8) and Muslims (0.7) conducted their marriage during the same age. Among the upper age at marriage groups who got married at 35 years and above the Hindus stands first (5.7%) followed by Muslims 2.7 and lowest among the Fishermen Christians (1.7%).

The preceding findings clearly confirm the differential age at marriage existing among girls and boys across three communities. Since the mean age at marriage of these women (19.8) is lower than the present age at marriage of girls in Kerala (21.9, 1981 Census). This factor would not have contributed appreciably in reducing their past fertility as compared to its present influence on the low fertility of women in Kerala.

Age at marriage and Fertility

Age at marriage of wives and husbands indicates a very pronounced inverse relationship with fertility behaviour, for the sample population as a whole and also among different religious groups. From the table 2.3 the range of difference in fertility between early age at marriage group and late marriage of women varies from 3.8 to 1.9. When the duration of marriage is controlled, more or less same trend is noticed among all the religious groups. In general, the highest fertility (3.8) is noticed in the age at marriage group of 13-15 years. When different age at marriage categories were examined, controlling the duration of married life of this women fertility is significantly lowest for the younger cohorts among all the three communities compared to the older cohorts. For the young cohorts in most of the age at marriage categories fertility is lowest for the Hindus, higher for the Muslims and highest for the Christians. But for the older cohorts it is once again lowest for the Hindus, followed by a higher fertility for Christians and highest for the Muslims in most of the age at marriage categories. Hence age at marriage differentially influenced the fertility of the younger and older cohorts of women among these communities (see table 2.3).

The husband's age at marriage also manifests a definite negative association with fertility for the population as a whole and also across the three communities. While the husbands who married at $\leq$ 19 years the fertility was lowest for the Hindus (3.6) highest for Christian Fishermen (4.6) and a medium level for Muslims (4.0). Interestingly, such cross cultural variations in fertility reduce to the minimum in significant level when marriage takes place at 30 and above. Among all the three communities, however, it continues to be lower for the Hindus and higher for the other two groups.

Table 2.3 : Mean live births according to the age at marriage of wife by the three religious groups and duration of married life

Age at marriage of wife	Hindus		Christians		Muslims		Total
	Duration of married life						
	≤10	11+	≤10	11+	≤10	11+	
≤ 12 years	2.0@	–	–	–	–	4.0@	3.0 (2)@
13 - 15 years	2.0	3.9	2.4@	4.1	2.0	5.1	3.8 (79)
16 - 18 years	1.9	3.5	2.6	5.1	2.2	4.5	3.5 (368)
19 - 21 years	2.0	3.2	2.4	4.2	2.0	4.5	2.7 (338)
22 - 24 years	1.8	3.1	1.5	3.6@	2.0@	2.3@	2.2 (149)
25 + years	1.6	2.8	1.3	2.0	-	-	1.9 (64)
Total	1.9 (317)	3.3 (299)	2.4 (117)	4.7 (116)	2.1 (65)	4.5 (86)	2.9 (1000)

@ Figures are less than ten in the columns.

According to the data given in the table 2.4, the range of ideal age at marriage for boys reported by an overwhelming proportion of the respondents in general and also all the three communities falls between 25-28 years. No doubt it varies significantly among the Christians on the one side and the Hindus and Muslims on the other. Surprisingly, the next largest proportion of 16.5 per cent of respondents reported still higher ages of 29 or more as the ideal age at marriage for boys. In this case significantly more Hindus (22%) compared to the Christians (6.4%) and Muslims (10.6%) wanted their children to marry very late. However, another 11 per cent of the respondents in general preferred an ideal lower age at marriage of 24 years or less. Under this category the Christian Fishermen constitute the largest proportion (26.6%) followed by a tenth of the Muslims and a negligible percentage of Hindus (5%).

Ideal Age at marriage of Boys and Girls

Table 2.4 : Percentage distribution of ideal age at marriage of boys across three religious groups

Ideal age	Hindus	Christians	Muslims	Total
≤ 20 years	0.3@	7.7	1.3@	2.2 (22)
21 - 24 years	5.0	18.9	8.6	8.8 (88)
25 - 28 years	72.9	67.0	79.5	72.5 (725)
29 + years	21.8	6.4	10.6	16.5 (165)
Total	100.0 (616)	100.0 (233)	100.0 (151)	100.0 (1000)

Ideal Age of Girls at Marriage

Table 2.5 : Percentage distribution of ideal age at marriage of girls across the three religious groups

Ideal age	Hindus	Christians	Muslims	Total
≤ 17 years	3.2	15.0	18.5	8.30 (83)
18 - 21 years	79.4	74.3	73.6	77.30 (773)
22 + years	17.4	10.7	7.9	14.40 (144)
Total	100.0 (616)	100.0 (233)	100.0 (151)	100.0 (1000)

At the aggregate level an overwhelming proportion of respondents preferred an ideal age at marriage of 18-21 years for girls. The same trend is more or less similar among the Christians and Muslims, but slightly higher among the Hindus. It is in line with the national policy on age at marriage of girls. Added to this another 15% of the respondents opted for still higher ideal age at marriage for girls (22 + years) and they are significantly more among the Hindus (17.4%) than among the Christians (11%) and Muslims (8%). It is also encouraging to note that only 7 per cent of the respondents preferred an age at marriage of 17 or less years. Such respondents are significantly more among the Christians (15%) and Muslims (18.5%) than among the Hindus (3.2%).

The preceding findings are encouraging among the Hindus and Muslims but not among the Fishermen Christians. If the reported ideal age at marriage of this couple is to guide the future behaviour of this parents, enough scope would be there to reduce birth rate further in future through the influence of higher age at marriage. But it cannot be confirmed similarly for the Fishermen Christians since they still opt for lower age at marriage for sons and daughters. Added to this, appropriate education and incentives may have to be introduced besides minimising the cost of marriage to translate the ideal age at marriage of parents into reality. This is because ideal age at marriage alone may not influence the actual age at marriage as there are other determinants involved.

Determinants of Age at Marriage

The concept of age at marriage cannot be understood fully unless the salient determinants of age at marriage are also taken into account, which is essential for planning appropriate interventions to manipulate future age at marriage for both girls and boys. Since the age at marriage of girls is mostly lower than the legally prescribed age at marriage, greater focus is given on determinants of age at marriage of girls. The selected salient factors of determinants of age at marriage considered here for discussion are (i) cost of arranging marriage including, total cost, item wise cost of dowry and ornaments, (ii) education of the wife, (iii) occupation of the wife, (iv) family income and various reasons for early marriage and late marriage.

Cost of Arranging Marriage

When the total cost of marriage expenses computed out of the cost involved in giving dowry, ornaments and other related expenses, it was found that the single largest proportion of 46 per cent of the respondents in the population as a whole spent Rs. 10,000 to 30,000 for the marriage of their daughters. Surprisingly, significantly more Christians (53%) followed by Hindus (47%) and Muslims (31%) spent so much for the marriage of their daughters. The second major proportion of 20 per cent of respondents, however, spent only Rs. 10,000 or less which again is highest among the Christians (31%) followed by Hindus (17%) and lowest among Muslims (14.5%). Another 16 per cent spent Rs. 30,000 to Rs. 50,000 for the marriage of their daughters. They constitute the highest proportion among the Caste Hindus (21%) followed by Muslims (11%) and lowest among the Fishermen Christians (8%). It is astonishing to note that 18 percent of the population in general spent Rs. 50,000 or more for celebrating the marriage of their daughters. They constitute the highest proportion of (44%) among the Muslims followed by (16%) Hindus and a negligible percentage of Fishermen Christians (8%).

Table 2.6 : Percentage distribution of respondents by total expenditure of marriage of daughter

Total expenditure	Hindus	Christians	Muslims	Total
≤ Rs. 10,000	17.1	31.2	14.5	19.9 (66)
10,001 - 30,000	46.7	53.2	30.9	45.6 (151)
30,001 - 50,000	20.6	7.8	10.9	16.0 (53)
50,001 +	15.6	7.8	43.6	18.4 (61)

Cross-cultural variations in the cost for conducting the marriage of daughters revealed that marriage is very expensive among the Muslims (54%) followed by the Caste Hindus (36.3%) and relatively less among the Fishermen Christians (15.6%) since they spent over Rs. 30,000 per marriage of daughters. Even the moderate expenditure of Rs. 10,000 to Rs. 30,000 per marriage is costlier for an ordinary family under the present economic difficulties. So much expenditure is incurred by 53 per cent of the poor Fishermen Christians followed by 31 per cent of the Muslims and 47 per cent of the Hindus. No doubt many of the Muslims can afford to invest higher amounts for celebrating the marriage of daughters as they are now better off with the newly acquired wealth from the gulf countries. But this is not true for most of the Fishermen Christians and a section of Hindus. These exorbitantly increasing cost of marriage of daughters is the most important determinant of early or late marriage compared to all other factors. It is not only an abnoxious custom in a welfare state but also can do deterioration of the status of women, neglect of female children and also even female infanticide. Thanks to the historical legacy of matriliny in Kerala, female infanticide is not practiced and the status of women is highest compared to other states, despite the mounting cost of marriage of daughters.

Determinants of Early Marriage of Girls

As determinants of early marriage of girls several reasons have been reported (see table 2.7). Generally the major reasons reported are: (1) marriage has to be arranged when parents are in an economically active position (45.8%), (2) keeping grown up girls in the family is a strain (43.1%), (3) to avoid risk of girls going astray (41.5%). The less frequent reason reported is that cinema going creates early sexual needs (10.9%). Among different caste groups significant variations have been observed for all these reasons. The Hindus reported less importance for early marriages as against 50 per cent of the fishermen Christians and muslims giving importance to early marriage. Among the Hindus not even a single reason has been mentioned by 50 per cent of the respondents. The reason extensively agreed to by the single largest proportion of the respondents (35.2%) is that marriage should be arranged early for the girls, when parents are in the active economic life. The least frequently reported reasons according to the Hindus and Christians are that cinema going creates early sexual needs but for the Muslims gave the lowest priority for the reason to avoid dowry (11.3%). Most of these factors were similarly identified by another two Indian studies (Mahadevan et al., 1986).

The three extensively reported reasons are to be given serious thought by the policy makers and administrators to minimise their influence on early age at marriage of girls. In this context unless the

Table 2.7 : Major reasons for arranging marriage of daughters earlier than 18 years in across three religious groups

Reasons	Hindus	Christians	Muslims	Total
To avoid dowry	8.6	24.5	11.3	12.7 (127)
To avoid risk of girls going astray	51.7	31.7	60.9	41.5 (415)
Keeping grown up girls in family is a strain	33.8	61.8	52.3	43.1 (431)
Marriage should be arranged when parents are in economically active position	35.2	64.4	60.3	45.8 (458)
Cinema seeing creates early sexual need	8.0	16.7	13.9	10.9 (109)
Pressure of relatives and neighbours	9.6	29.6	19.9	15.8 (158)
Religious conventions	7.8	25.3	34.4	15.9 (159)

Note : Totals are not equal to 100% multiple reasons are given.

cost of marriage is brought down by introducing several practical measures, parents will continue to insist on early age at marriage of girls when they are in active economic life. The other two reasons are born out of the fear of parents about the girls possibly indulging in premarital sex. To prevent this risk, sex education may be introduced right from middle school level onwards in order to teach the boys and girls about the adverse consequences of premarital sex. It may also be extended to all dropouts through the adult education programme. Since the relatives give pressure to conduct early marriages they should also be exposed to the idea of importance of late marriage through population education and adult education programmes. The adverse effect of cinema as promoting sexual feeling at early ages is a dangerous trend. Therefore certain guidelines may be issued to the cinema producers and censoring agencies to minimise the present excessive and vulgar trends in films.

Determinants of Late Marriage

Determinants of late marriage (Table 2.8) are not extensively reported as in the case of early marriage. In the population as a whole the highest percentage (20.6) delayed marriage because the required amount of dowry could not be raised. For another 11.7 per cent marriage was delayed because suitable alliances were not readily available. All other reasons according to their importance are: (1) waiting for completion of education (8.8%), (2) no matching horoscope (7.3%), (3) waiting for job (6.4%), and (4) problem in adjustment with husband (1.5%). Among the different caste groups variations have been widely observed on these aspects. According to the present data, more Hindus have been practicing late marriage compared to the other two groups. All the three communities uniformly cited the most important reason as the difficulty in raising dowry on time – 23.5 per cent for the Hindus, 20.5 per cent for Muslims and 12.9 for Fishermen. another 10-14 per cent of the Hindus reported three reasons viz., absence of suitable alliance, non-agreement of horoscope, waiting for completion of education. No doubt another 8 per cent of the Hindus also delayed their marriage in order to get a job. A similar proportion of Muslims also delayed the marriage in order to get suitable alliance and for the completion of education, besides waiting to get a job before marriage (6.6%). But none of these reasons were similarly important for the Christian Fishermen.

All these factors and a few more were reported in three other recent studies in Kerala (Mahadevan, 1985 & 1986; Zachariah, 1983). Their findings also more or less agree with the present result. Hence it is confirmed that these factors could be made use of in the formulation of new policies and interventions to increase the female age at marriage in our country.

Educational Status and mean Age at Marriage of Wife

Education is one of the major factor that leads to the delay in marriage of couples, especially wives. Findings from several studies significantly revealed that education generally has a strong and positive relationship with age at marriage (Mahadevan, 1986; Audinarayana, 1985; Whelpton et al., 1966; Driver, 1963; U.N. 1961). From the present data (Table 2.9) it is also confirmed that a positive relationship between education and age at marriage is observed.

Table 2.8: Reasons for late marriage: Major reasons for arranging daughters marriage above 20 years

Reasons	Hindus	Christians	Muslims	Total
Horoscope not matching	10.9	0.9	2.7	7.3 (73)
Suitable alliance was not available	14.6	4.3	11.3	11.7 (117)
Dowry could not be raised	23.5	12.9	20.5	20.6 (206)
Waited for completion of education	10.4	4.3	9.3	8.8 (88)
Waited for job	8.0	2.2	6.6	6.4 (64)
Adjustment with husband	2.0	0.4@	1.3@	1.5 (15)

Note: Totals are not equal to 100% because multiple reasons are given.

For the total population age at marriage varies from 18.3 - 20.9 between illiterate to highly educated women. The overall observations from this data show that Hindus have higher age at marriage compared to the Muslims and Christians. For the younger and older cohorts of all the religious groups, only Christians showed the lowest age at marriage among the illiterates, but for the Muslims, lowest age at marriage was observed for those who studied from class one to 4th standard and among the Hindus for those people who studied from 5-7 classes. At the same time highest age at marriage was observed among those who attained college education, irrespective of all the religious groups. But their number is negligible among the Muslims and Christian fishermen and more among the Hindus. Thus education automatically increases the age at marriage among all the communities and also for the young and old women. But the increase in age at marriage is more pronounced in the case of younger cohorts of women in all the communities. This difference may be due to higher proportion of the young women being educated and also marrying late compared to older women. Even the illiterate young women married at slightly higher ages than the older women. This may be on account of general upward shift taking place on the age at marriage as a result of overall social changes in the institution of marriage.

Table 2.9 : Mean age at marriage according to education of wife, religion and duration of married life

Education of wife	Hindus		Christians		Muslims		Total
	Duration of married life						
	≤10	11+	≤10	11+	≤10	11+	
Illiterate	20.2	19.0	17.7	17.3	18.8@	16.8	18.3 (147)
1 - 4	22.1	18.7	18.3	17.6	17.5@	16.5	18.7 (225)
5 - 7	20.5	18.4	18.7	17.0	18.6	17.3	18.8 (208)
8 - 10	21.0	19.3	20.8	19.7	19.0	17.4	20.0 (350)
College educated	21.5	20.9	21.2@	20.0@	21.8@	19.0	20.9 (59)
Total	21.0 (317)	18.9 (299)	18.9 (117)	17.9 (116)	18.9 (65)	17.0 (86)	19.3 (1000)

@ Sample is less than ten.

Occupational Status of Wife and Age at Marriage

Occupational status of a person may also influence age at marriage directly and indirectly. In general, people with better occupations have higher age at marriage. The present data also to a certain extent confirmed the same trend. The age at marriage is lowest for the lower occupational status group like labourers (18.7), still higher among petty business women (18.9), and housewives (19.2), and the highest (21.7) among the educated and employed women in the population as a whole. A more or less similar trend is noticed among the Muslims and Hindus, but an inconsistent trend is noticed among the Christians.

Table 2.10 : Mean Age at Marriage and Occupational Status of Wife, religion and duration of married life

Occupation	Hindus		Christians		Muslims		Total
	≤10	11+	≤10	11+	≤10	11+	
Labourers	20.1	18.4	19.5	17.0	19.0@	17.0	18.7 (151)
Petty businessmen	23.4@	18.4	18.7@	18.4	20.0@	15.5@	18.9 (50)
Housewives	21.0	19.0	18.8	18.1	18.7	17.2	19.4 (769)
Educated employees	23.2	22.3@	-	17.0@	22.3@	16.0@	21.7 (30)
Total	21.0 (317)	18.9 (299)	18.9 (117)	17.9 (116)	18.9 (65)	17.0 (86)	19.3 (1000)

@ Sample less than ten.

While considering the mean age at marriage between the young and old cohorts of women across the three cultural groups, it is uniformly seen that the young cohorts of women who follow all the four major categories of profession married at higher ages than the older cohorts of women. Under most of the categories of occupation, Hindu women whether young or old, married at higher ages than the other two communities. Between the latter two communities there is no consistent trend in this regard. Thus education coupled with occupation together cause substantial increase in age at marriage in most of the communities, but such differences are however, not statistically significant, except among the Hindus.

Income and Age at Marriage

Economic status of the family marginally confirms a positive association with mean age at marriage in the population as a whole. But the range of difference was from 19.2 to 20.1 for the lower and upper income categories. A more or less similar trend is noticed among all the communities and also within each community for young and old cohorts of women. The increase in age at marriage from lower to the higher income group is more pronounced among the younger cohorts than the older cohorts among all the three communities.

Table 2.11 : Mean age at marriage of wife and family income

Income	Hindus		Christians		Muslims		Total
	≤10	11+	≤10	11+	≤10	11+	
≤10,000	20.9	19.0	18.8	17.4	18.7	17.2	19.2 (660)
10,001 to 20,000	21.2	19.0	18.5	18.8	19.0	16.9	19.6 (279)
20,001 +	22.0	18.7	24.3@	18.5@	21.8@	16.0@	20.1 (61)
Total	21.0 (317)	18.9 (299)	18.9 (117)	17.9 (116)	18.9 (65)	17.0 (86)	19.3 (1000)

@ Sample less than ten.

Taking education, occupation and economic status of the family and their influence on mean age at marriage, greater influence is seen with the impact of education compared to the other two socio-economic variables. Therefore, the existing difference in education among the three communities might be a major determinant of the variation in age at marriage noticed among these groups. Obviously the Hindus followed by the Muslims are relatively more educated than the Fishermen Christians. Among the Hindus, however, age at marriage did not reveal much difference across among the different caste groups. Similar is the case with respect to family type.

THREE

SOCIO-ECONOMIC STATUS AND FERTILITY

Socio-economic development of the major communities in Kerala varied not only in the present but also historically. Before 1900 the socio-economic status of the Hindus of the upper caste was far better than the rest of the communities. This trend has now very much changed since independence because of several policies and reforms introduced by the successive governments in Kerala. In this context the land reform measures adopted rigorously by the communist governments preceded the several changes accomplished among the Scheduled castes and tribes, Christians and Muslims. They were the major beneficiaries of the land reform because the land was owned mostly by the upper Caste Hindus in the past.

Subsequently, the wide spread facilities created for education initially by Christians, the upper caste Nairs and Backward Ezhavas provided with spread education first among Christians and the upper castes and only later to the rest of the population. Added to this the Caste Hindus and the Christians also had the early advantage of getting new occupation within and outside Kerala because of their early attainment of extensive education. The migration of the people in search of employment outside the state provided them with an added advantage of earlier attainment of modernization and economic emancipation compared to other communities.

Now, however, this trend has become a common feature for all the communities since 1970's. Hence the upper Caste Hindus and Christians became economically better off compared to the Muslims and the Harijans. Of course this does not apply to the Fishermen Christians who continue to be illiterate and poor, despite the social changes that swept through Kerala during this century. These historical differential opportunities of development and the concurrent social change that took place among these communities during the remote particularly and the recent past contributed to the different levels of socio-economic development among the Hindus, Christians and Muslims in Kerala. Hence it is appropriate to see their historical differences from the empirical data given below. They include: Family structure, Type of house, Electrification of house, Education, Occupation, Economic status and opportunity cost and their relationship on fertility behaviour.

1) *Family Structure*: Family structure, Type of house and Housing condition compose one of the major determinants of socio-economic status of the people. Family structure has been trichotomised here into joint family, transitional family and nuclear family. The transitional family is in a state of transition from joint family to nuclear family, which includes nuclear family with certain adult male or female dependents but not two couples. In the past, however, joint family was universal perhaps till the end of 19th century. The pace of nuclearization of families increased after 1947, when several land reforms and wealth tax measures were introduced by the communist and successive governments in Kerala and also as a result of emigration of people from Kerala to far-off places. The trend of change noticed below (see table 3.1) in the wide spread prevalence of nuclear family (61%) as against only 17 per cent transitional family and 22 per cent joint family, manifest the present family structure in the population as a whole. When family structure is examined across different cultural groups, the nuclear family is significantly more among the fishermen Christians (74%) than among the Hindus (57.3%) and Muslims (57.6%). interestingly, Hindus and Muslims have similar proportion of nuclear families, transitional families and joint families. It is obvious that more Christians have taken to nuclear families because they are all mostly the fisher folk and live in independent households. This is more or less true for the other Christians also because of the modernization, most Christians established new households soon after their marriage. The tendency for adult dependency seems to be less among the Christians and also among the Muslims.

According to the table 3.2, fertility behaviour is directly related to the changing structure of the families in the population as a whole, across different communities and among young and old couples. Significant differences in fertility are noticed between joint and nuclear families in most of the communities and also among couples with less than or equal to 10 years of married life and over 11 years of married life. The fertility differences continue to persist among the three communities for the young and old couples belonging to joint, transitional and nuclear families. Both under joint and nuclear families also the Christians manifest the highest fertility followed by the Muslims and the Hindus. It is obvious that fertility is highest among the Christians because an overwhelming proportion of them live in nuclear families compared to the other two communities. Therefore, greater prevalence of the nuclear families and its pronatalist influence among the Christians may be a contributory factor for the highest fertility noticed among the Christians. Thus the hypothesis confirmed here in that the characteristics of nuclear families contribute to high fertility, irrespective of communities and duration of married life. One obvious reason noticed here for the high fertility in the nuclear families and low fertility in joint families is on account of relatively more young people (≤10 years of married life) seen in joint families and more older cohorts of women seen in nuclear families. It is also natural that privacy will be more in nuclear families and hence the frequency of sex may be more there, which can contribute to high fertility. On the other hand, in joint families, there may be restrictions, voluntary or involuntary separation for the spouses which may naturally reduce their frequency of sex (Nag, 1962, Mahadevan, 1985-86). These factors together may contribute to the existing differences in fertility between the joint and nuclear families.

Table 3.1 : Percentage distribution of respondents according to the Type of Family by the three religious groups

Type of family	Hindus	Christians	Muslims	Total
Joint family	25.1	14.5	22.5	22.2 (222)
Transitional family	17.6	11.2	19.9	16.5 (165)
Nuclear family	57.3	74.3	57.6	61.3 (613)
Total	100.00 (616)	100.0 (233)	100.0 (151)	100.0 (1000)

Table 3.2: Mean live birth according to the Type of Family, Religion and duration of married life

Type of family	Hindus		Christians		Muslims		Total
	Duration of married life						
	≤10	11+	≤10	11+	≤10	11+	
Joint family	1.6	3.0	2.0	4.5	1.6	3.6@	2.1 (222)
Transitional family	1.9	4.1	2.2	4.6	2.0@	4.0	3.1 (165)
Nuclear family	2.0	3.3	2.7	4.8	2.6	4.9	3.3 (613)
Total	1.9 (317)	3.3 (299)	2.4 (117)	4.7 (116)	2.1 (65)	4.5 (86)	2.9 (1000)

@ Sample less than ten.

Type of House

Generally, socio-economic status variables have shown a negative association with fertility. According to the present data it is confirmed that type of house variable shows significant difference with fertility behaviour for the population as a whole, and among all the religious groups.

Table 3.3 : Percentage distribution of respondents according to the Type of Hours by the three religious groups

Type of houses	Hindus	Christians	Muslims	Total
Kutcha	42.4	64.4	34.4	46.3 (463)
Semi-pucca	40.9	27.9	49.7	39.2 (392)
Pucca	16.7	7.7	15.9	14.5 (145)
Total	100.0 (616)	100.0 (233)	100.0 (151)	100.0 (1000)

Among the total sample of single largest proportion of the people (46.3%) are living in Kutcha houses, followed by semi-pucca (39.2%) and pucca (14.5%). According to religion-wise classifications, significantly more Christians live in Kutcha houses (64.4%), followed by Hindus (42.4%) and Muslims (34.4%). Regarding pucca houses, they are more among the Hindus (16.7%) followed by Muslims (15.9%) and least for Christians (7.7%). It reveals the differential economic status of the population as a whole. Thus relatively more Hindus are found to be living in prosperous houses than Muslims and Christians. But between the latter two communities, relatively more Muslims live in better houses than the Christians.

Table 3.4 : Mean live birth according to Type of House, Religion and Duration of married life.

Types of House	Hindus		Christians		Muslims		Total
	Duration of married life						
	≤10	11+	≤10	11+	≤10	11+	
Kutcha	2.1	3.4	2.6	4.7	2.2	4.8	3.1 (463)
Semi-pucca	1.8	3.4	2.1	5.3	2.1	4.5	2.9 (392)
Pucca	1.8	3.1	1.3	3.0	1.8	3.8	2.6 (145)
Total	1.9 (317)	3.3 (299)	2.4 (117)	4.7 (116)	2.1 (65)	4.5 (86)	2.9 (1000)

Housing conditions of the family showed a more or less definite negative association with fertility behaviour (table 3.4). For the population as a whole the level of fertility varies from 3.1 to 2.6 for those who are living in Kutcha and Pucca houses. A similar trend was noticed among all the caste groups. When the duration of married life is controlled, variations have also been observed among different caste groups. For the young cohorts of women, fertility showed a uniformly negative association with type of house in all the three communities. When the mean live birth of the younger cohorts is considered across the three communities, it is lowest among the

Hindus followed by the Muslims and highest among the Christians for the Kutcha houses. But in case of semi-pucca houses also, the Hindus have the lowest fertility and the other two communities showed similar mean live births. In the case of pucca houses, the differences in fertility have narrowed down among them to an almost equal level. In the case of older cohorts also, a similar negative association is noticed with respect to type of house in all the three communities. The relationship is more pronounced in the case of Muslims followed by the Hindus but a slightly inconsistent association is noticed for the Christians.

Electrification of House

Table 3.5: Percentage distribution of respondent according to electrification of house by the three religious groups

Electrification	Hindus	Christians	Muslims	Total
Not electrified	43.8	64.8	37.1	47.7 (477)
Electrified	56.2	35.2	62.9	52.3 (523)
Total	100.0 (616)	100.0 (233)	100.0 (151)	100.0 (1000)

Table 3.6 : Mean live birth according to electrification of house, Religion and Duration of Marriage

Electrification	Hindus		Christians		Muslims		Total
	Duration of marriage life						
	≤10	11+	≤10	11+	≤10	11+	
Not electrified	2.0	3.4	2.6	4.6	2.2	5.2	3.1 (477)
Electrified	1.9	3.3	2.1	4.7	2.0	4.1	2.8 (523)
Total	1.9 (317)	3.3 (299)	2.4 (117)	4.7 (116)	2.1 (65)	4.5 (86)	2.9 (1000)

For the general population nearly half (52%) live in electrified houses (table 3.5). However, among the three communities a significantly higher population of Muslims (63%) live in electrified house followed by Hindus (56%) and Christians (35%). Normally the electrification of the house may show a clear trend in fertility behaviour (table 3.6). When electrification of house is examined in relation to fertility behaviour, the population as a whole, across the three communities and also within the communities for different age cohorts, fertility is less in electrified as against non-electrified houses. However, the difference is more conspicuous for Muslims only, except for the older cohorts of Muslims and young cohorts of Christians the fertility difference is not statistically significant between the electrified and non-electrified houses. In this context, since only one third of Christian houses are electrified, a special efforts may have to be given by the government to provide electricity for the houses of the fishermen community on a priority basis for the sake of fertility control and also for their own welfare.

Education and Fertility

Education constitutes the most important and powerful social variable that explains fertility behaviour all over the world. It is a variable that constitutes the modernization of people. It is also a component of social stratification. Historically, many studies have shown the persisting strong inverse relationship between education and fertility (Kiser, 1960; Driver, 1963; Agarwala, 1966; Blake, 1967; Minkler, 1970; Mahadevan, 1979). However, educational level is normally very low among women in general in most of the developing countries, and for men, it is comparatively better. In India, according to 1981 census, the literate men constitute 46.7 per cent as against 24.9 per cent of women. Of course, in developed countries, women are extensively educated compared to developing countries. Generally, educational level manifests a negative association with fertility behaviour in case of both developed and developing countries. From the late nineteenth century, this relationship is diminishing or even disappearing in some low developed fertility countries (U.N., 1973). According to a cross nation World Fertility Survey, low level of education is not a factor that depresses fertility.

For Kerala the largest single factor that contributed to fertility decline in recent times has been education. The literacy level of the population as a whole in Kerala as per 1981 census was 69 per cent as against the all India figure of 36 per cent. But women's literacy rate was 64.5 per cent in Kerala as against 24.9 for India.

Table 3.7: Percentage distribution of the education of wife and religion

Education	Hindus	Christians	Muslims	Total
Illiterate	9.6	27.5	15.9	14.7 (147)
1 - 4	17.2	35.2	24.5	22.5 (225)
5 - 7	24.5	13.7	16.6	20.8 (208)
8 - 10	39.9	20.2	37.7	35.0 (350)
College education	8.8	3.4	5.3	7.0 (70)
Total	100.0 (616)	100.0 (233)	100.0 (151)	100.0 (1000)

Table 3.8 : Percentage distribution of the Education of husband and religion

Education	Hindus	Christians	Muslims	Total
Illiterate	6.0	36.0	4.6	12.8 (128)
1 - 4	15.9	16.7	27.8	17.9 (179)
5 - 7	25.5	17.2	28.5	24.0 (240)
8 - 10	39.5	25.8	29.8	34.8 (348)
College education	13.1	4.3	9.3	10.5 (105)
Total	100.0 (616)	100.0 (233)	100.0 (151)	100.0 (1000)

The present data reveal that literates constitute 85 per cent in the sample population as a whole. However, literacy level varies according to the religious groups. They are highest among the Hindus, followed by Muslims and somewhat less among Fishermen Christians, which may not be the pattern among non-Fishermen Christians. Regarding the level of education of women a more or less similar trend is noticed among the Hindus, Christians and Muslims. The fact, those who have attained class Vth and above are much higher among the Hindus compared to Muslims and Christians, but for those who have studied up to class 1st to IVth, a significantly higher proportion is seen among the Christians followed by Muslims and the Hindus (see table 3.7).

The educational level of the husbands in general in the population revealed that 87 per cent of them are literates. When considered community wise, the level of education of the husbands shows a similar trend. While the Christians constitute the highest proportion of illiterates, the same category among the Hindus and Muslims are similar (6 and 5 per cents respectively). Nevertheless, the highest educated people, i.e., from class VIIIth and above, are significantly more among the Hindus compared to the Muslims and Christians. For women also a similar trend is noticed. But on the educational level from class I to VII, the Muslims men out number the Hindus and Christians. But such a trend is not there for women (see table 3.8).

Educational Status and Fertility of Wife and Husband

Educational attainment of husband and wife indicates a definite inverse relationship with fertility behaviour for the population as a whole. According to the present data a negative association between education and fertility has been significantly observed both for the husbands and wives, irrespective of religious groups. Hence the hypothesis referred to earlier has been fully confirmed. The range of difference in fertility between the illiterates and higher educated women in general varies from 3.9 to 1.2. The corresponding difference in fertility of men was 3.9 to 2.4. Thus this relationship was more pronounced among the wives as compared to husbands (see table 3.9)

When the duration of marriage is controlled, a similar trend is noticed among the religious groups. Among the young illiterate group ($\leq$ 10 years) and older women (11+ years) fertility is uniformly and significantly lower among the Hindus compared to the Christians and Muslims. A similar trend was observed for the men of these communities. When educational level increases from class I to VII, similar trend was observed for both wives and husbands. As the education further grows from class VIIIth onwards fertility was higher for younger and older women of the Hindus compared to Christians and Muslims. These findings show that higher education beyond class eight causes rapid decline in fertility more among Christian Fishermen and Muslim women than Hindus. No doubt it is also important in reducing fertility among Hindus as well. But in case of husbands no such significant difference was observed from class eight onwards also. Regarding highest level of education it is revealed that the fertility is lowest among the Fishermen Christians, both for younger and older groups followed by Hindus and Muslims.

Taking all the preceding findings together, we may confirm that education is a major antinatalist factor, which, of course reduces fertility differentially among different religious groups. The present findings in general confirm to the other earlier studies conducted in India (Rele and Kanitkar, 1980; Mahadevan, 1979; George, 1973; Driver, 1963; and U.N., 1961). But the present study has not only discussed its influence among population in general but also derived deeper into different caste and religious groups, which is an advancement compared to the earlier studies. These findings evidently support the urgent necessity for providing encouragement, including incentives, to the high fertility backward communities like the fishermen, the Muslims and the Harijans to control their fertility along with other low fertility communities.

Occupational Status

Occupational status of a person influences fertility behaviour directly and indirectly through education and age at marriage. In general, higher occupations need higher education, which in turn may postpone the age at marriage, and this leads to low fertility. Women employed outside the home normally would manifest a low level of fertility compared to those not employed outside the home, even when their socio-economic status remain same. According Limananda (1983), the case of females "Working outside the hom.

Table 3.9 : Mean live birth according to the education of husband and wife, religion and duration of marriage

Education of husband & wife	Hindus				Christians				Muslims				Total	
	Husband		Wife		Husband		Wife		Husband		Wife		Husband	Wife
	Duration of marriage													
	≤10	11+	≤10	11+	≤10	11+	≤10	11+	≤10	11+	≤10	11+		
Illiterate	2.6	3.5	2.4	4.0	2.7	6.1	2.7	5.9	2.5	6.2	3.4	5.3	3.9 (128)	3.9 (147)
1 - 4	2.1	3.5	1.9	3.4	3.2	4.8	2.7	5.1	2.2	4.5	1.8	5.0	3.5 (179)	3.5 (225)
5 - 7	2.1	3.5	2.0	3.3	2.4	3.9	2.6	4.1	2.3	5.2	2.1	4.9	3.1 (240)	2.9 (208)
8 - 10	1.8	3.2	1.9	3.2	1.9	3.6	1.8	3.1	1.9	3.4	1.8	3.1	2.4 (348)	2.4 (350)
College education	1.7	3.0	1.6	2.8	1.2	2.6	1.2	2.0	2.2	3.4	2.4	2.7	2.4 (105)	1.2 (70)
Total	1.9 (317)	3.3 (299)	1.9 (317)	3.3 (299)	2.4 (117)	4.7 (116)	2.4 (117)	4.7 (116)	2.1 (65)	4.5 (86)	2.1 (65)	4.5 (86)	2.9 (1000)	2.9 (1000)

for pay before marriage is as important as educational attainment in providing women a chance to enlarge their circle of life, to gain more freedom in managing their own level".

Table 3.10 : Percentage distribution of respondents according to occupation of wife and religion

Occupation of wife	Hindus	Christians	Muslims	Total
Labourers	16.7	17.1	5.4	15.1
Petty business	3.1	10.3	4.6	5.0
Housewives	76.8	71.7	85.4	76.9
Educated employees	3.4	0.9@	4.6@	3.0
Total	100.0 (616)	100.0 (233)	100.0 (151)	100.0 (1000)

@ Frequency less than ten.

Table 3.11 : Percentage distribution of husbands according to occupation and religion

Occupation of husband	Hindus	Christians	Muslims	Total
Labourers	44.4	20.2	38.4	37.9 (379)
Rural artisans	6.8	0.9	-	4.4 (44)
Fishermen	-	58.0	-	13.6 (136)
Business	15.4	7.3	27.8	15.4 (154)
Government employees	23.4	9.0	14.6	18.7 (187)
Employed in Gulf countries	10.0	4.6	19.2	10.0 (100)
Total	100.0 (616)	100.0 (233)	100.0 (151)	100.0 (1000)

In the present data showing in table 3.10, an overwhelming percent of women (76.9%) in general are engaged in household duties, followed by labourers (15.1%) and small scale business people (5%). In case of educated employees, they constitute only a negligible percent (3%) of the population as a whole. Among the different religious groups, the percentage of housewives is highest among the Muslims (85.4%), followed by Hindus (76.8%) and slightly less among the Christians (71.7%). In case of labourers, Muslims constitute the lowest percentage (5.3) compared to the other two groups (Hindus, 16.7%; Christians, 17.2%). More or less same trend is noticed for educated employees also, but among Christians and Muslims their number is very negligible. These findings by and large confirm the poor status of affairs on occupational mobility among women in the study area. Nevertheless it cannot be projected for Kerala state as a whole, because occupational mobility of women is comparatively better than in rest of the country.

According to table 3.11 the occupational status of men reveal that the single largest percentage of them are engaged as labourers (37.9%). On the basis of religion the labourers are found more among the Hindus (44.5%) followed by Muslims (38.4%) and Christians (20.2%). At the same time, fishing, which is the traditional occupation of the Christian Fishermen is the occupation 13.6 per cent of the total population and 58 per cent among the Christians themselves. On the whole, 18.7 per cent of husbands were engaged in government jobs, 15.4 per cent in business and 10 per cent of them are working in Gulf countries. On the basis of religion a significantly high percentage of them are Muslims (19.2%), followed by the Hindus (9.7%) and the Christians (4.7%). On the whole, only a minority of population are engaged as rural artisans (4.4%). Rural artisans are significantly more among the Hindus and negligible among Christians (0.9%) and nil among Muslims.

The preceding findings confirm that a significantly high proportion of the Muslims (61.8%) have moved to higher and new occupations followed by the Hindus (48.5%) and the Fishermen Christians (20.7%). It is fascinating to note that occupational mobility coupled with migration is significantly more among the Muslims (19%), followed by Hindus (9.7%) and the Fishermen Christians. This occupational mobility would have certainly contributed to improvement in economic status and modernization of the menfolk on a differential basis among the populations studied here. The same trend is also noticed in the general population except for the Christians. According to P.R.G (1983), the largest population of menfolk who migrated from Kerala to Gulf countries are the Muslims followed by Christians and lastly Hindus. Between the husbands and wives, occupational mobility is extensive among the husbands as compared to wives. However, it cannot be concluded that women have less occupational mobility as seen here because in the sample population the women employed outside the home would not have been enumerated due to their non-availability. Nevertheless, the occupation is still to a certain extent synonymous with that of the religion and caste despite the mobility in occupation noticed during the recent past. Muslims by and large work as manual labourers, do business or are employed in services. Christians engage in almost all categories of work as also the Hindus.

Considering the influence of differences in occupational status with wives and husbands together it is confirmed that the couple employed in non-traditional occupations have the lowest fertility. It is also true for the husbands employed in Gulf countries. This hypothesis is fully confirmed, irrespective of the cultural groups and control of the duration of married life of the women (see table 3.12 and 3.13). While examining the differences of fertility across the different occupations held by the womenfolk, the highest fertility is noticed for those who engage in petty business and labourers. Among men, the fishermen, artisans and also labourers manifest the highest fertility. Community-wise trend of older cohorts of women indicates that women employed as labourers among the Muslims and petty business women of the Hindus showed the highest level of fertility. But among the Christians, a more or less uniform level of high fertility is noticed among almost all occupational categories except the labourers. However, among the young cohorts such variations are not very conspicuous. Considering the occupational status of menfolk across the three communities for the same period of married life, fertility is highest for the labourers, Muslims, fishermen Christians and artisan Hindus. Hence men and women engaged in traditional occupations continue to manifest high fertility in all the communities.

Table 3.12 : Mean live birth according to occupation of wife, religion and duration of marriage

Occupation of wife	Hindu		Christians		Muslims		Total
	Duration of marriage						
	≤10	11+	≤10	11+	≤10	11+	
Labourers	2.3	3.4	2.3	3.9	2.7@	5.8	3.1 (151)
Petty business	2.4@	3.6	2.4@	5.0	1.0	4.5	3.8 (50)
Housewives	1.9	3.3	2.4@	5.0	2.1	4.5	2.9 (769)
Educated	1.7	3.1@	-	5.0@	2.0	2.7@	2.4 (30)
Total	1.9 (317)	3.3 (299)	2.4 (117)	4.7 (116)	2.1 (65)	4.5 (86)	2.9 (1000)

@ Sample less than ten.

Economic Status

Economic status historically showed an inverse relationship to fertility, though it is undergoing changes in the modernized and industrialised countries in the recent past (Saksena, 1973; U.N., 1973; Freedman et al., 1959; Sinha, 1957; Whelpton and Kiser, 1946-1958). The economic status of the sample population was measured in terms of the annual income of the family. The major source of income was either salaries or daily wages, business and other sources, such as from landed property and house rent and money from Gulf countries. According to the present study (table 3.14), the highest proportion of the people in general (66%) secured a total income of Rs. ≤10,000 per annum, followed by 28 per cent who were earning Rs. 10,001 to 20,000. The remaining 6 per cent alone have an annual income of Rs. 20,001 and more. Among the different religious groups, the Christian fishermen constitute the highest percentage of (74.3%) poor people with an annual income of Rs. ≤10,000 followed by Muslims (68.2%) and Hindus (62.3%). In the case of middle income groups, the Hindus constitute greater percentage (31%), followed by Muslims (24.5%) and the Christians (23%). Regarding the highest economic group, the Muslims (7.3%) and Hindus (7%) constitute a more or less similar proportion but only a negligible percentage of Fishermen Christians have an annual income of Rs. 20,000 and more. At the same time, however, the number of Muslims and Christians were very few in the upper income category. From these findings it is confirmed that the Fishermen Christians are economically poorest among all the religious groups. No doubt this trend may not truly reflect the non-Fishermen Christians who are concentrated in the Central Travancore and Cochin region and who are economically far better off than even their Hindu counterparts.

Table 3.13 : Mean live birth according to occupation of husband, religion and duration of marriage

Occupation of husband	Hindus		Christians		Muslims		Total
	Duration of marriage						
	≤10	11+	≤10	11+	≤10	11+	
Labourers	2.0	3.4	1.8	3.7	2.3	5.3	3.0 (379)
Rural artisans	2.2	4.3	-	2.5@	-	-	3.2 (44)
Fishermen	-	-	2.8	5.9	-	-	4.1 (136)
Business	1.9	3.4	2.0	3.8@	2.6	4.6	2.9 (154)
Government employees	1.9	3.1	1.4@	2.8	2.1	3.1	2.5 (187)
Employed in Gulf countries	1.7	2.9	1.5@	3.2@	1.7	3.4	2.2 (100)
Total	1.9 (317)	3.3 (299)	2.4 (117)	4.7 (116)	2.1 (65)	4.5 (86)	2.9 (1000)

@ Sample less than ten.

Table 3.14 : Percentage distribution of family income and religion

Income	Hindus	Christians	Muslims	Total
≤10,000	62.3	74.2	68.2	66.0 (660)
10,001/- 20,000/-	30.7	22.8	24.5	27.9 (279)
20,001/- +	7.0	3.0@	2.3	6.1 (61)
Total	100.0 (616)	100.0 (233)	100.0 (151)	100.0 (1000)

The level of fertility on the basis of economic status was hypothesised to have an inverse relationship, but the findings did not confirm this trend. For the population as a whole fertility is highest among the middle income groups (3.1) followed by the lowest economic group 2.9 and the highest economic status group 2.3. A similar trend is noticed among the older cohorts of Hindus and Christians, but among similar groups of Muslims, fertility is more among the lower status groups. Among the younger cohorts the mean live birth is lowest among the Hindus and Muslims and lower income groups of the Christians. Hence a more less positive curvilinear relationship was observed between income and fertility behaviour. Among the Christians and Muslims low fertility is noticed in the upper economic status group but their number is very negligible in their respective columns (see table 3.15)

Opportunity Cost

For measuring the opportunity cost perceived by the respondents, a composite index was developed using a few sensitive dimensions of the opportunity cost (Babbie, 1983). The dimensions considered are that children reduce the opportunity for the parents to (i) take rest, (ii) seek pleasure, (iii) reading and learning facility, (iv) take treatment, (v) properly look after children and (vi) better the educational career. Several other items considered for the construction of index could not be used because of their strong intercorrelation among themselves. However, though these items were related to one another, they have a separate identity. The logical validity (face validity) of the items were examined before they have been finally selected. The items selected also showed variation in their manifest behaviour when correlated with fertility. These items were classified dichotomously into two categories viz., important and unimportant. For each item, similar score of one to unimportant and two to important were assigned under each dimensions of the opportunity cost. The cumulative score range was calculated for all the items and they were once again classified into three equal groups which have been designated as low, medium and high opportunity categories. This tripartite classification of opportunity cost index was finally correlated with fertility behaviour.

Table 3.15 : Mean live birth according to family income, religion and duration of marriage

Income	Hindus		Christians		Muslims		Total
	Duration of marriage						
	≤10	11+	≤10	11+	≤10	11+	
≤10,000	2.0	3.2	2.4	4.3	2.2	4.6	2.9 (660)
10,001 20,000	1.8	3.7	2.5	5.5	1.9	4.5	3.1 (279)
20,001 +	1.9	2.8	1.3@	3.3@	1.1@	3.8@	2.3 (61)
Total	1.9 (317)	3.3 (299)	2.4 (117)	4.7 (116)	2.1 (65)	4.5 (86)	2.9 (1000)

@ Number of cases are less than 10 in these columns.

Out of the six items of the opportunity cost considered here, four items were found to be important to a significant proportion of population. According to their order of importance, difficulty to take treatment is ranked as first (51.4%) followed by absence of rest (50.6%) and problem of looking after children (47.8%) and inconvenience caused to leisure time activities (40%). The problem resulting from restrictions of educational opportunities, however, did not figure as a major item. It is retained as an item because the literacy level of Kerala is over 70 per cent according to 1981 census. In examining the same across the three communities a slight difference is noticed for different items. For Muslims and Christians, the number one item remains the difficulty to take treatment but for the Hindus, the principal item is the problem of getting rest. The second important item for the Muslims and Christians happened to be the problem of looking after children and for the Hindus the difficulty experienced for taking treatment. The third important problem seemed to be the difficulty in getting rest for Muslims and Christians and the constraints of looking after children for the Hindus. These items were more or less similar for the Muslims and Christians but much less among the Hindus. The fourth problem uniformly found for all the three communities is the difficulty to get time to enjoy life. The preceding differential inter-community trend noticed on dimensions of opportunity cost also correspondingly agree with their existing different levels of fertility. Since the Hindus have low fertility, the problem of opportunity cost is relatively less among them when compared to the other two high fertility communities.

The levels of opportunity cost perceived by the population in general showed a definite negative association with fertility behaviour. Those who perceived very high problem of opportunity cost have very low mean live births of 2.2 as against 3.8 of those who have perceived it as very low. While examining the same across three communities and among different cohorts of women, similar trend is noticed. Thus the hypothesis confirmed here is that increase in perception of different opportunity costs progressively reduces the fertility significantly, irrespective of the community background and the duration of married life of the mothers.

Consideration of the specific socio-economic status variables together confirmed that couples with better socio-economic status manifested significantly lower fertility as against their counterparts who were at the lower strata of the socio-economic hierarchy. It is true for the Muslims, Christians, Hindus and the young and old couples. Nevertheless, improvement in socio-economic status among women, particularly with respect to their education, showed pronounced decline in fertility as against the same conditions prevailing among their husbands. Since the Fishermen Christians and the Muslim women have poor educational status compared to the Hindu women, urgent attention may have to be given through non-formal education to improve their social status and level of modernization.

Table 3.16 : Percentage distribution of respondents by different dimensions of opportunity costs.

Dimensions of opportunity costs	Hindus	Christians	Muslims	Total
No rest	46.3	57.9	56.9	50.6 (506)
Seeking pleasure	34.3	50.2	47.0	39.9 (399)
Unable to read or spend time for gaining knowledge	9.3	0.9	7.9	7.1 (71)
Difficult to take treatment	45.8	61.8	58.3	51.4 (514)
Difficult to get time to look after children	40.1	61.4	58.2	47.8 (478)
Could not go for education	6.5	0.4	3.3	4.6 (46)

Note: Totals are not equal to 100%, multiple reasons are given.

Table 3.17 : Mean number of live birth according to the opportunity costs index

Opportunity costs Index	Hindus		Christians		Muslims		Total
	≤10	11+	≤10	11+	≤10	11+	
Low	2.3*	3.8*	2.9*	5.5*	2.6*	5.1*	3.8* (358)
Medium	2.2	3.3	2.9	4.7	2.7	5.0	3.4 (183)
High	1.7*	2.8*	1.7*	3.2*	1.7*	3.0*	2.2* (459)
Level of* significance	1%	1%	1%	1%	1%	1%	1%

FOUR

VALUE OF CHILDREN

The concept of value of children has become prominent in fertility theory and research during the middle 1970's but this macro theme encompasses diverse concepts and refers to several kinds of empirical studies (Berelson, 1976; Fawcett, 1972, 1977; Schultz, 1973). Perceptions of the value of children were treated as intervening variables to explain fertility through socio-economic change. The perceptions are influenced by structural features of the society in which the individual lives and his personal experiences. These structural factors included socio-economic status, cultural influence and sex roles. The impact of socio-economic factors has been a dominant concern in research on perceptions of the value of children in developing countries (Fawcett, 1983). Several cross cultural studies have been conducted with different focus in several Asian countries which have revealed that several dimensions of value exist in Most of these countries for valuing children (Bulatao, 1980; Fawcett, 1977; Lee and Kim, 1977; Arnold et al., 1975). They are social, economic cultural and psychological dimensions. These findings indicate that where children have economic or practical value in the household, these benefits dominate the way parents perceive the satisfaction of children. In some Asian societies, cultural factors favouring large families seem to have different roots. For example, in Indonesia, the positive cultural value of a "busy household" is regarded as a significant factor in the preference for large families (Darroch, Meyer and Singarimbun, 1981; Meyer, 1981). The evidence does suggest a broad cultural influence on the perceived value of children in the Philippines (Arnold et al., 1975, Bulatao, 1975). All these studies in developing and developed countries have shown a moderate strong relationship between some measures of the perceived satisfaction and cost of children and various measures related to family size and the practice of birth control (Arnold et al., 1975; Chang, 1979; Deven, 1977; Kagiteibasi and Esmer, 1980). A few other Indian studies given more emphasis on the old age security value

(Mahadevan, 1986; Cain, 1981, Vlassoff and Vlassoff, 1980). From all these studies it is confirmed that value of children is a major determinant of fertility. In the light of preceding findings of earlier studies it is hypothesised for the present study that the greater the value attached to the children/sons, the higher will be the fertility.

Dimensions of Value of Children (Sons)

According to the present data we have identified several dimensions of value of children, especially sons. They are economic, social, cultural and psychological values of the respondents. Among all the nine dimensions of the value of children, four of them were found to be more important for an overwhelming proportion of the total population. Those values are: Existing children need company (77.9%), Economic support during old age (74.6%); Salvation of parents (72.3%) and physical support in the family (71.5%). About half of the respondents give importance to values like; more sons will lead to better economic position (58.6%) followed by traditional lineage (52.5%). Another 35.7 per cent of the people have given importance to the need to dominate powerfully in village social life, 24.2 per cent of them have been given prominence to the inheritance of family property. The least frequently reported value (13.4%) that: "Sons bring more dowry to the family".

In the religion-wise classification, a similar trend was observed about the major items discussed earlier. Among the three religious groups, Muslims (75%) and Christians (71.2%) have given highest priority to the first value, i.e., "Existing children need company", but among the Hindus, highest preference goes to "salvation for parents after death" (83.3%). The least frequently reported value for the Muslims (13.3%) and Hindus (12.0%) was "sons bring more dowry" and among Christian Fishermen (14.2%) the lowest importance is assigned to the value of children inheriting family property. However, almost all the dimensions of value of children cross cultural variations in terms of their prevalence have been observed. Out of the extensively confirmed four dimensions of value of children, a significantly higher proportion of Hindus have manifested these values, followed by the Muslims and the Christians (See table 4.1).

Table 4.1 : Percentage distribution of respondents according to the importance given to different dimensions of value of Son(s)

Dimensions Value of Son(s)	Hindus	Christians	Muslims	Total
Economic support during old age	80.5	61.8	70.5	74.6 (746)
Inherit family property	26.6	14.2	30.4	24.2 (242)
For the physical support in the family	73.6	70.5	65.0	71.5 (715)
Dominate powerfully in the village social life	40.9	22.6	35.1	35.7 (357)
More sons will lead to better economic position of the family	64.9	48.5	48.5	58.6 (586)
Existing children need Company	81.2	71.2	75.0	77.9 (779)
Salvation for parents after death	83.3	48.1	64.9	72.9 (729)
Provide traditional links (lineage)	61.6	36.2	40.7	52.5 (525)
Sons bring more dowry	12.0	17.2	13.3	13.4 (134)

Value Dimensions and Fertility

On the basis of Table 4.2 fertility differences resulting out of significant influence of five dimensions of value of children have been noticed in the population as a whole. According to their order of importance, the following dimensions of the value of children have increased the level of fertility from 0.4 to 0.7 child when the parents gave importance to these values; they are: "Sons are needed to bring more dowry; more sons will improve the economic position of family; they are necessary for physical support to the family; old age economic support; and existing children need company". Out of these five major pronatalist dimensions of value of children, four of them are found to be highly important across the three communities.

they are: Sons are important to bring more dowry; more sons will lead to better economic position of family; sons are prominent important to give physical support to the family and provide old age security. Among these four major dimensions of value of children, the first item is important among the Christians and Muslims for increasing their level of fertility (Christians, 1.5 child and Muslims 0.8), but it could increase the fertility among Hindus only 0.2 baby which is significantly less (significant at 1%) compared to its influence among the other two communities. The second factor 'son will lead better economic position' is also highly important to the Christians (1.1) followed by Hindus and Muslims. The third factor is equally important among all the three communities. Fourth significant factor (old age security) is the most important factor among the Hindus, because it increases their fertility by 0.6 child and it is equally important among the Christians and Muslims (0.4). However, considering all the nine value except 'sons bring more dowry' significant difference are observed among the fertility of Hindus. But all other factors showed similar trend among the Muslims and Christians. In the light of the preceding discussions, three dimensions of value of children are found to be universally important to the population as a whole for increasing their fertility (Economic values and value on physical ability). A fourth value dimension (to bring more dowry) is found important only among the two communities, viz., Christians and Muslims but not for Hindus, and a fifth one 'Existing children need company', is significant only for the Hindus, but not among the Christians and Muslims. The other four dimensions are not conspicuous and consistent in their pronatalist influence among the Muslims and Christians. Out of the three crucial dimensions of value of children which were found among the three communities, only physical support to the family and one economic value of children were found important among the Muslims, while several dimensions of value of children were increasingly found important among the Hindus and some extent Christians.

Value of son(s) Index

For measuring the overall importance of value of son(s) a composite index was constructed. For this purpose the various dimensions of value of children considered are: Old age economic support, inheritance of family property, physical support in the family, need to dominate in the village social life, better economic position of the family, existing children need company, salvation for the parents after death, traditional lineage and sons bring more dowry.

Table 4.2 : Mean live birth according to value dimensions of son(s)

Value dimensions	Hindus		Christians		Muslims		Total	
	1	2	1	2	1	2	1	2
Economic support during old age	2.7	2.1	3.7	3.3	3.5	3.1	3.1 (746)	2.7 (254)
Inherit family property	2.9	2.4	3.2	3.6	3.5	3.4	3.1 (242)	2.9 (758)
For physical support in the family	2.8	2.0	3.8	3.0	3.6	3.0	3.1 (715)	2.4 (285)
Dominate powerfully in the village social life	2.9	2.3	3.7	3.5	3.4	3.5	3.1 (357)	2.9 (643)
More sons will lead to better economic position of the family	2.7	2.2	4.1	3.0	3.6	3.2	3.1 (586)	2.6 (414)
Existing children need company	2.6	2.0	3.6	3.3	3.5	3.4	3.0 (779)	2.6 (221)
Salvation for the parents after death	2.6	2.0	3.8	3.3	3.5	3.3	3.0 (723)	2.9 (277)
Provide traditional lineage	2.9	2.0	3.3	3.5	3.2	3.7	3.1 (525)	2.9 (475)
Sons bring more dowry	2.8	2.6	4.8	3.3	4.2	3.4	3.6 (134)	2.9 (866)

Note: 1 = Important; 2 = Unimportant.

All those dimensions of value of children that showed significant influence on fertility behaviour were selected for developing the index. All such items were classified as important and unimportant in relation to value of children. For the unimportant item a score of one was assigned and for the important item two was given. The cumulative score of all the dimensions of value of children was added up and a score range was prepared which was equally divided into low, moderate and high value categories. These items were correlated with fertility in order to know the differential degree of importance given to value of children by the respondents. The distribution of respondents in general according to the degree of importance given to the value of children (see Table 4.3) was largest under the moderate category (42%). People who attribute high or less value were almost equal in their proportions (high 30%, less 29%). When these distributions were examined across three communities, the largest proportions of Muslims and Hindus gave the highest value for sons for moderate importance (46% and 42%) and the Christians less important (43%) in this category. While the second largest proportion of respondents among the Hindus (36%) and Muslims (32%) were highest in their value for sons, Christians (40%) manifested moderate value for sons. However, a quarter of Hindus (23%) only did not attribute any importance to sons as against a significantly higher proportions among the Christians (43%) and Muslims (30.9%).

The degree of value of children based on the index showed in Table 4.4 a direct relationship with fertility behaviour on the population as a whole. The range of increase in mean live birth increased from 2.5 to 3.2 when the importance given to the sons increased among the respondents. These differences are statistically significant (Significant at 1% level). When the same thing is examined across the three communities, a similar trend is noticed. However, the variations in fertility behaviour among the respondents of these communities who gave least value or highest value varied significantly. Those who gave least value had the lowest fertility among the Hindus (2.0) followed by Muslims (2.9) and the Christians (3.1). A similar trend is noticed among these communities when they attributed highest value to the sons. With regard to the moderate value also a similar trend is noticed. Hence the hypothesis fully confirmed here is that the concept of value of sons in general is important for all the population, irrespective of their cultural background and of course, with certain differences. Nevertheless, value of son(s) differentially increases the fertility among the three communities.

Table 4.3 : Percentage distribution of respondents by value of children based on index

Index	Hindus	Christians	Muslims	Total
Less value	22.6	43.0	30.9	28.8 (288)
Moderate	41.7	40.3	46.3	41.6 (416)
High value	35.7	16.7	31.8	29.6 (296)

Table 4.4 : Mean number of live birth according to value of children index

Index	Hindus	Christians	Muslims	Total
Less value	2.0*	3.1*	2.9*	2.5* (288)
Moderate	2.7	3.8	3.4	3.1 (416)
High value	2.8*	3.9*	3.6*	3.2* (296)
* Level of significance	1%	1%	1%	1%

FIVE

BREASTFEEDING AND FERTILITY

Breastfeeding is a major proximate determinant of fertility behaviour according to several studies summarized by Bongaarts and Potter (1983). A number of studies have demonstrated a strong correlation between breastfeeding and the duration of amenorrhea and between breastfeeding and the birth interval at the individual level (Prema and Raveendranath, 1982; Huffman, 1981; McNeily, 1979; Bongaarts, 1978). The mechanism of its influence on fertility behaviour is through the lactational amenorrhea period that extends or reduces with the duration of breastfeeding. Breastfeeding is the best form of nutrition for infants and its contraceptive effect has been the principal regulator of human fertility. Further, lactation has an inhibiting effect on ovulation and thus increase the birth interval and reduces natural fertility. However, studies from India, Egypt, Chile and from several developed countries suggest that lactational amenorrhea shortens among women who introduce supplementary feeding at an early age during infancy (Prema and Raveendranath, 1982).

Breastfeeding is universal in the study population. The mean duration of breastfeeding for the population as a whole is 15.1 months. It is 14.9, 15.7 and 15.3 for the Hindus, Christians and Muslims respectively. An overwhelming proportion (81%) of mothers breastfed their babies several months beyond a one month period (see Table 5.1). However, 19 per cent of the mothers breastfed their babies for a very short period of less than a month. Their number is significantly more among the Hindus (20.6%), followed by the Christians (17.2%) and the Muslims (13.9%). Since the Hindus, by and large, have lower mortality and are better off compared to the other two communities in the study area, they would have discontinued breastfeeding earlier for the sake of beauty and other such reasons. It is unfortunate that the poor Fishermen Christians do not universally breastfeed their children for a long period. This would have affected the health of their babies. The nutritional status of the Muslims is not poor compared to the other two groups, and they have breastfed the largest number of children (86%) for a long period. The general norm of breastfeeding ranges up to 2 years and less in all the three communities, and the same is more among the Muslims followed by the Christians and the Hindus. This period is demographically more important because the amenorrhea period will fall within this range of duration of breastfeeding. Therefore, breastfeeding would have contributed to the suppression of ovulation at least slightly over 50 per cent of the population for a long period of time. The mean amenorrhea period for the population as a whole is 7.9 months and among the three communities, it is 7.0, 9.7 and 8.5 for the Hindus, Christians and Muslims respectively. Another 16.5 per cent of the population breastfeed their babies beyond two years of time, which in all probability would not have any demographic importance, because the amenorrhea period may not be prolonged beyond two years of time and the cultural taboos on avoidance of sex after delivery may not exist during this time to benefit the fertility reduction.

Table 5.1 : Percentage distribution of respondents according to duration of breastfeeding by the three religious groups

Breastfeeding (in month)	Hindus	Christians	Muslims	Total
Breastfeed less than a month	20.6	17.2	13.9	18.8 (188)
1 - 24	61.2	67.9	74.2	64.7 (647)
25 - 36	13.2	13.7	9.2	12.7 (127)
37 +	5.0	1.2	2.7	3.8 (38)
Total	100.0 (616)	100.0 (233)	100.0 (151)	100.0 (1000)

Table 5.2 : Mean live birth according to duration of breastfeeding, religion and duration of married life

Duration of breastfeeding (in months)	Hindus		Christians		Muslims		Total
	Duration of married life						
	≤10	11+	≤10	11+	≤10	11+	
Breastfed less than a month	1.1 (110)	1.8 (17)	1.2 (35)	1.4 (5)	1.1 (17)	2.0 (4)	1.2 (188)
1 - 24	2.4 (174)	3.5 (203)	2.9 (74)	5.0 (84)	2.5 (44)	4.7 (68)	3.4 (647)
25 - 36	2.4 (29)	3.7 (52)	2.7 (8)	4.3 (24)	1.7 (3)	4.4 (11)	3.4 (127)
37+	2.2 (4)	2.7 (27)	-	4.3 (3)	2.0 (1)	4.3 (3)	2.9 (38)
Total	1.9 (317)	3.3 (299)	2.4 (117)	4.7 (116)	2.1 (65)	4.5 (86)	2.9 (1000)

Note Generally in the previous tables figures are not given in the brackets to facilitate the easy reading. However, under this section figures are given for identifying the variations in each group.

Generally the duration of breastfeeding manifested an inverse relationship with fertility behaviour in the population as a whole for the women who breastfed their babies for a period of one month and beyond (see Table 5.2). However, the women who breastfeed for less than one month also showed low fertility; it is largely because most of them happened to be younger women, who have only just begun their child bearing; this could be seen when we controlled the duration of married life. The above trend is seen in all the communities as well. Thus prolonged breastfeeding acts as an antinatalist force in all the communities and the population as a whole. Nevertheless, its influence is more among the older couples.

Postpartum amenorrhea period

The mean postpartum amenorrhea period for the population as a whole is 7.9 months and among the three communities it is 7.0, 9.7 and 8.5 for the Hindus, Christians and Muslims respectively. These findings in no way explain the influence of amenorrhea, on low, medium and high fertility levels of the Hindus, Muslims and Christians, because the Hindus, who have the lowest fertility, also have the lowest duration of postpartum amenorrhea period as against the Christians who have the highest fertility and show the longest duration of amenorrhea period when examined within one year and over one year periods. According to Table 5.3 it is seen that an overwhelming proportion of the population (79%) and also similar proportion of the Hindus (83%) and the Muslims (80%) have a duration of one year or less amenorrhea periods. But significantly lower percentage of Christians (66%) have an amenorrhea period of only one year or less. Those who have a year or more of amenorrhea period constitute only 17 per cent for the population as a whole and 11 and 19 per cent respectively among the Hindus and Muslims, as against significantly more proportion of Christian women (27%) who have an amenorrhea period of over one year. When the duration of amenorrhea period is further examined for the shorter intervals of time it can be seen that a single largest proportion of the total population (41%) and also in all the communities manifest a short duration of 1-4 months amenorrhea period (see Table 5.1). Another quarter of the population and also for the different communities showed an amenorrhea period of 9 to 12 months. All other categories of duration of amenorrhea the trend is not seen extensively among the population as well as all the communities.

Postpartum amenorrhea and fertility

In table 5.4, fertility behaviour in relation to amenorrhea period showed a somewhat negative association in the population as a whole. It also showed a negative association among the three communities and within the communities for the young and older cohorts of women. However, the peak period of fertility is manifested for the women who have an amenorrhea period of 1-8 months. In most of the cases fertility is seen to decline when the amenorrhea period extends to nine months and beyond.

Table 5.3 : Percentage distribution of respondents according to the period of amenorrhea by the three religious groups

Amenorrhea period	Hindus	Christians	Muslims	Total
Period not specified	4.7	7.3	1.3	4.8 (48)
1 - 12 months	82.9	65.7	80.2	78.6 (786)
13 + months	12.4	27.0	18.5	16.6 (166)
Total	100.0 (616)	100.0 (233)	100.0 (151)	100.0 (1000)

Table 5.4 : Mean live birth according to amenorrhea period by religion and duration of married life.

Duration of amenorrhea period in months	Hindus		Christians		Muslims		Total
	Duration of married life						
	≤10	11+	≤10	11+	≤10	11+	
Not specified	1.0 (19)	1.7 (10)	1.5 (12)	1.4 (5)	1.0 (2)	—	1.3 (48)
1 - 4 months	1.9 (148)	3.5 (140)	2.8 (34)	5.0 (30)	2.4 (35)	5.1 (27)	3.0 (414)
5 - 8 months	2.5 (41)	3.3 (38)	2.6 (10)	4.9 (14)	2.1 (10)	4.9 (14)	3.2 (127)
9 - 12 months	2.3 (75)	3.2 (70)	2.5 (30)	4.8 (35)	1.9 (10)	4.2 (25)	3.1 (245)
13 -24 months	1.4 (30)	2.9 (31)	2.1 (27)	4.5 (26)	1.5 (8)	4.0 (17)	2.7 (139)
25 + months	1.3 (4)	2.1 (10)	1.5 (4)	4.1 (6)	-	2.7 (3)	2.4 (27)
Total	1.9 (317)	3.3 (299)	2.4 (117)	4.7 (116)	2.1 (65)	4.5 (86)	2.9 (1000)

Avoidance of sex after delivery

Normally in Kerala as a whole, sex is taboo for 56 days after delivery. But it is prolonged or reduced depending upon the couple and the communities concerned. In the present study, population as a whole, sex is avoided after delivery for a period of eleven weeks. However, Muslims on an average avoid it for 12 weeks, followed by the Hindus (11.2 weeks) and Christians (9.9 weeks). This trend of differential duration of avoidance of sex after delivery may be an indicator showing their differential influence on fertility behaviour. While the Christians have the shortest duration of avoidance of sex they also have the highest fertility which speaks about the pronatalist influence of this factor among a high fertility community. The table 5.5 given in the appendix also more or less confirms an inverse relationship between duration of sex avoidance and fertility behaviour in the population as a whole and also for the older and young cohorts of women in most of the communities. Therefore, it is a natural and culturally acceptable factor which may have to be reinforced through population education for the benefit of low fertility.

Table 5.5 : Percentage distribution of respondents according to duration of sex avoided after delivery by three religious groups

Duration of sex avoided in weeks	Hindus	Christians	Muslims	Total
≤ 4 weeks	2.6	11.6	1.3	4.4 (44)
5 - 8 weeks	21.7	27.9	18.5	22.7 (227)
9 - 12 weeks	61.8	48.5	54.4	57.6 (576)
13 + weeks	13.9	12.0	25.8	15.3 (153)
Total	100.0 (616)	100.0 (233)	100.0 (151)	100.0 (1000)

SIX

BIRTH INTERVALS AND FERTILITY

One of the most important factors that will control the fertility of women is the maintenance of longer interpregnancy interval. According to Bongaarts (1983), married and fecund women reproduce at a rate inversely related to the average duration of the birth interval. Short birth intervals are associated with high fertility and vice-versa. Birth intervals in human population offer an interesting, fruitful and at the same time intriguing area of scientific enquiry (Srinivasan, 1980). Birth intervals can be categorised into two broad types: the closed interval, which is the interval between the successive live births of a women and the open interval, which is the interval from the date of the last live birth to the date of survey.

There is a growing body of literature which provides more direct evidence for a positive association between the duration of breastfeeding and the length of birth interval. A birth interval can be divided into three main components (1) postpartum amenorrhea, (2) menstruating interval and (3) gestation period. The length of the birth interval is primarily determined by the duration of breastfeeding and the use of contraception (Bongaarts and Jain, 1980).

According to the present study, birth intervals (closed and open) were taken as independent variables and their influence on fertility behaviour was studied. Hence we considered here closed birth intervals as intervals between last child and last but one child. Open birth interval means the interval from the date of the last live birth to the date of survey.

Closed Birth Interval

Mean duration of closed birth interval constitutes only 25.5 months for the population as a whole. However, it slightly varies between the Muslims (27.8 months) and non-Muslims (25 months), when the proportion of distribution of population according to different duration of closed birth interval is considered (Table 6.1). It is highest (30%) for the duration ranging from 13 to 24 months followed by 37 months and more (25%) and another quarter of them had the duration of 25 to 36 months. There is only a negligible 4 per cent of population which had a closed birth interval of one year or less. Considering the ideal duration of closed birth interval of three years and more, it is noticed only among a quarter of the population and in fact, an overwhelming proportion of population (75%) had experienced shorter birth interval of less than 3 years. This duration of birth interval significantly varied across these communities only from 2 years and more. For the longer duration of birth interval of two years and more a significantly high proportion of population is seen among the Muslims as against the Christians and Hindus. However, the longest duration of open birth interval is found extensively among the Hindus as against the Muslims and Christians. Since the duration of closed birth interval is not sufficiently long for the population, intensive population education has to be mounted to increase the inter-birth interval in order to improve the maternal and child health status, besides making it a positive family planning measure.

The duration of closed birth interval is negatively associated with fertility behaviour for the population as a whole (Table 6.2). The same trend is noticed among the three communities and also for the younger and older cohorts of women. Therefore, the duration of closed birth interval would have contributed to the differentials and changes in fertility of at least 25 per cent of the population. For this category of population closed birth interval would have substantially contributed to their low fertility (3.2 children) with the population as a whole. Thus closed birth interval is a major determinant of low fertility of a quarter of population in general; but not for the major segment of the population.

Open Birth Interval

Mean duration of open birth interval in the population as a whole is 28 months. However, it varies between the Christians (23.3 months) and the non-Christians (Hindus 28.7; and Muslims 29.5 months). The longest duration of open birth interval ranging from six years and above (which is a determinant of fertility behaviour) is extensively seen among the largest proportion of population (32.8%). It also significantly varies between the Hindus (36.7%) and non-Hindus (26%). The longest duration of open birth interval was more among the Hindus. It may not be due to secondary sterility, but may be because of the highest rate of family planning adoption status. However, open birth interval is extensive among the older cohorts of women compared to the young. On the other hand, shorter duration of open birth interval of one to two years also varies among the three communities, but the shorter birth interval of less than two years is highest among the Christians (43.8%) followed by the Hindus (31.8%) and the Muslims (28.5%). These differential durations of open birth interval therefore might contribute to the existing difference in fertility among these communities, because the Hindus, who have the lowest fertility and the largest proportion of women have a longer duration of open birth interval. On the other hand the largest proportion of Fishermen Christian women have the shortest duration of open birth interval, and they also have the highest fertility. However, such distinct differences are not visible among the Muslims.

Table 6.1 : Percentage distribution of respondents according to closed birth interval and religion

Birth interval	Hindus	Christians	Muslims	Total
1. N.A.	18.5	14.6	12.0	16.6 (166)
2. ≤12 months	4.7	2.2	2.5	3.8 (38)
3. 13 – 24 months	28.9	33.9	30.5	30.3 (303)
4. 25 – 36 months	21.8	30.0	25.2	24.2 (242)
5. 37 + months	26.1	19.3	29.8	25.1 (251)
Total	100.0 (616)	100.0 (233)	100.0 (151)	100.0 (1000)

Though for the population as a whole, open birth interval did not show a definite influence on fertility behaviour, it is because a higher proportion of older women are there with the longest duration of open birth interval. However, a clear trend has emerged when the duration of married life is controlled. Among all the three communities, for the younger and older cohorts of women, fertility is lowest for the couples with longest duration of birth interval. Thus an inverse relationship is more or less visible under all the three communities for the younger and older cohorts. Hence open birth interval has differentially influenced the fertility of the three communities, taking into consideration the inverse relationship of all the three groups and the differential proportion of women in the short and long open birth interval categories.

Table 6.2 : Mean live births according to closed birth interval, religion and duration of marriage

Closed birth interval	Hindus		Christians		Muslims		Total
	Duration of marriage						
	≤10	11+	≤10	11+	≤10	11+	
1. N.A.	1.00 (103)	1.00 (11)	1.00 (30)	1.00 (4)	1.00 (16)	1.00 (2)	1.00 (166)
2. 12 months	2.5 (13)	3.8 (16)	2.5 (2)	5.3 (3)	-	5.1 (4)	3.7 (38)
3. 13–24 months	2.4 (86)	3.6 (92)	2.9 (42)	4.9 (37)	2.7 (20)	5.1 (26)	3.4 (303)
4. 25–36 months	2.4 (66)	3.4 (68)	2.9 (30)	5.3 (40)	2.1 (16)	4.7 (22)	3.4 (242)
5. 37 + months	2.2 (49)	3.2 (112)	2.6 (13)	4.0 (32)	2.3 (13)	4.0 (32)	3.2 (251)
Total	1.9 (317)	3.3 (299)	2.4 (117)	4.7 (116)	2.1 (65)	4.5 (86)	2.9 (1000)

Note: Generally in most of the tables figures are not given in the brackets to facilitate the reading of the table. However under this section figures are given in the brackets for identifying the variation in each group.

Table 6.3 : Percentage distribution of respondents according to open birth interval and religion

Open birth interval	Hindus	Christians	Muslims	Total
24 months	31.8	43.8	28.5	34.1 (341)
25 - 48 months	17.4	20.6	28.5	19.8 (198)
49 - 72 months	14.0	9.0	16.5	13.3 (133)
73 + months	36.8	26.6	26.5	32.8 (328)
Total	100.0 (616)	100.0 (233)	100.0 (151)	100.0 (1000)

Table 6.4 : Mean live birth according to open birth interval, religion and duration of marriage

Open birth interval	Hindus		Christians		Muslims		Total
	Duration of marriage						
	≤10	11+	≤10	11+	≤10	11+	
24 months	1.9 (173)	3.6 (23)	2.5 (80)	6.5 (22)	2.1 (35)	5.1 (8)	2.5 (341)
25 - 48 months	2.0 (82)	3.7 (25)	2.4 (26)	5.2 (22)	2.1 (25)	5.2 (18)	2.9 (198)
49 - 72 months	1.9 (46)	3.2 (41)	2.3 (7)	4.4 (14)	1.8 (5)	4.3 (20)	2.9 (133)
73 + months	1.5 (16)	3.3 (210)	2.0 (4)	3.9 (58)	-	4.1 (40)	3.3 (328)
Total	1.9 (317)	3.3 (299)	2.4 (117)	4.7 (116)	2.1 (65)	4.5 (86)	2.9 (1000)

SEVEN

CONTRACEPTION AND FERTILITY

Every society has in some way attempted to exercise some control over the number, quality or characteristics of its population. Family planning is used in the sense of deliberate birth control including contraception, abortion and sterilization. It is the voluntary planning and action of individuals and or couples to limit the number of children they want. Family planning methods can be described as the devices, drugs, substances and techniques employed to delay or prevent births. The practice of contraception induces a decrease in the monthly risk of conception; thus, instead of its natural value, fecundity will have a lower residual value that is a function of the effectiveness of the contraceptive method used (Leridon, 1977).

According to Bongaarts (1983), contraception is one of the important proximate determinants of fertility. Contraceptive prevalence varies widely among countries; it is less than 10 per cent in a number of developing countries, and it reaches near 80 per cent in some developed societies. Sterilization has undergone a rapid increase to substantial levels in a number of countries (Rose and Huber, 1982). A world wide review (Lubell and Frischer, 1980) estimates that out of 90 million couples sterilized for contraceptive purpose by 1978, China alone contributes to 36 million, India 22 million and the United States 12 million. In India today, there are perhaps more than 10 million couples who do not want to have more than two children (ORG, 1976).

Kerala is reported to be one of the most successful states in India with respect to family planning practice. In 1980, about 30 per cent of the currently married women were effectively protected from pregnancy through the services of the official family planning programme. Zachariah (1983) recently conducted a study in Kerala which reported that 28 per cent of the currently married women were sterilized or had husbands who were sterilized. Further, acceptance of family planning is estimated to have caused a reduction of about 10 points in the crude birth rate by 1980, which also agrees fairly well with the findings of sample registration system (SRS, 1981).

Table 7.1 : Percentage distribution of respondents according to family planning adoption status and the three religious groups

Family planning adoption status	Hindus	Christians	Muslims	Total
Non-adopters	21.8	42.9	29.8	27.9 (279)
Permanent adopters	57.0	46.8	45.7	52.9 (529)
Temporary adopters	21.2	10.3	24.5	19.2 (192)
Total	100.0 (616)	100.0 (233)	100.0 (151)	100.0 (1000)

According to the present data (Table 7.1), an overwhelming (72%) proportion of population have been using any one of the permanent or temporary methods for birth control at the time of this study. Among the total adopters, 53 per cent of them adopted permanent methods like sterilizations. Another 19 per cent continue to use temporary methods for prevention of birth or for the purpose of delay in birth. On the basis of religion, significant differences are observed across the three groups. The level of adoption of the Hindus constitute the highest percentage (78.2) followed by the Muslims (70.2%) and the Fishermen Christians (57.1%). This significant difference in acceptance of contraception across these communities constitutes a major determinant of the highest fertility noticed among the Fishermen Christians, lowest fertility among the Hindus and a moderate level for the Muslims. Hence, this hypothesis has been confirmed in this population.

The information on use of various contraceptives indicated that tubectomy is the widely prevailing method. The World Fertility Survey (1980), result also similarly confirmed that, in the recent trends sterilization as a contraceptive method, and particularly voluntary female sterilization, is the most widely used contraceptive method in the world. About 95 million women depend on this method to control their fertility (Population Report, 1985). Among the total adopters, 63.4 per cent of them have currently adopted tubectomy, but in the case of vasectomy only 10 per cent of them have accepted it so far. This might be due to several reasons and notably because many problems are associated with vasectomy, and the tubectomy is convenient during delivery time. Adoption of different methods according to religious background reveal that an overwhelming percentage (72.2) of Fishermen Christians are using tubectomy as a method of birth control, followed by the Hindus (62%) and Muslims (58.5%). In the case of vasectomy highest percentage of adopters (10.8%) are seen. Among the Hindus followed by Christians (9.8%) and Muslims (6.6%). At the same time, adoption status of temporary methods like coitus interruptus and safe periods together constitute the highest percentage (14.3%) at the aggregate level. Among the Muslims, 21 per cent of the adopters are practicing this method followed by Hindus (13.9%) and Christians (10.5%). The main reasons for the highest percentage of adoption of temporary methods by the Muslims (see table 7.1), is that some of them believe sterilization is a sin and some religious leaders are also against this method. Under these circumstances the only method of contraception is self-control including coitus interruptus. Most of the Muslims are aware of this coitus interruptus. Several religious leaders like Mullah and Maulavis also gave information about this method and supported it while opposing sterilization. At the same time artificial contraceptives, viz., Nirodh, IUD and Pills are being used by 9 per cent, 1.8 per cent and 1.5 per cent respectively by the population as a whole. It is interesting to note that a tenth of the Hindus and Muslims have adopted Nirodh as against only a half (5.3%) among the Christians. Why is such difference noticed among the Christians. It may be because they live mostly in huts and single room houses. As far as IUD is concerned it is highest among the Christians (2.3%) followed by the Muslims (1.9%) and Hindus (1.7%). Surprisingly, Pill use is more common among the Muslims (2.8%) followed by the Hindus (1.7%) and nil among the Christians. The preceding differential use of temporary methods of contraceptives provide several ideas for strengthening the differential promotion of these methods among these communities. In the face of opposition to sterilization by the Muslim priest, it is appropriate to concentrate more on temporary methods among them. Subsequently, when motivation for contraception increases they can be persuaded to accept sterilization.

Similarly, there is no point in insisting upon the promotion of Nirodh among Fishermen Christians and such others who live in single room house or huts where facilities for its use is limited. Since more Muslims have come forward to accept Pills it may be given a fair trial because of less objection to this method. Thus the present strategy on promotion of contraceptives may be changed on the lines mentioned above to expedite the promotion of family planning programme among all the communities.

The effect of birth control on natality may be defined in a simple way from a theoretical or modeling point of view; it is the number of births averted owing to use of a family planning method. In practice in a real population - the concept is not so simple, since one is never sure what the behaviour of users would have been if the method had not been available to them. There are many reasons for this uncertainty, the most important being that the population of family planning "acceptors" is never completely similar to that of non-acceptors (Leridon, 1977). Generally fertility level is negatively associated with contraceptive behaviour. Most of the studies conducted in India revealed that adopters of permanent methods of contraception had higher fertility in comparison to the current users of temporary methods and non-users (Mahadevan, 1986; Reddy, 1982; ORG, 1970). The present data also confirms more or less the same results. According to the present study (table 7.2), in general, temporary adopters have low fertility (2.3) compared to non-adopters (2.6) and permanent adopters (3.4). The non-adopters are having less than 0.5 children compared to adopters of family planning method. At the same time the difference is 1.1 children between the temporary and permanent method of adopters.

These findings revealed that the temporary adopters are going in for spacing and not for termination. Further, their adoption is demographically effective because they have attained only 2.3 live births. Out of them living children will be either two or even less. The demographic effectiveness of permanent adopters is not very great, because they have already attained 3.4 live births and among them at least three children will be living. Nevertheless, even adoption of sterilization with three children is a big achievement compared to the live birth of sterilized people in other parts of the country. However, it is surprising to note that a very high proportion of people with 2.6 live birth have not accepted any family planning methods so far. In comparison between the three religious groups, when their duration of married life is controlled for the temporary adopters, except for the younger cohorts of Hindus, all others are showing the lowest fertility. Among the younger cohorts of the Hindus, lowest fertility was observed among non-adopters but the difference is not significant. In the case of older cohorts of the Hindus same level of fertility was noticed among all the three groups. At the same time younger and older cohorts of Christians and Muslims,

Table 7.2 : Mean live births according to family planning adoption status, religion and duration of married life

Family planning adoption status	Hindus		Christians		Muslims		Total
	Duration of married life						
	≤10	11+	≤10	11+	≤10	11+	
Non-adopters	1.5*	3.3*	2.3*	5.3*	1.9*	5.4*	2.6* (279)
Permanent	2.5*	3.3*	3.0*	4.7*	2.7*	4.8*	3.4* (529)
Temporary	1.6	3.3	1.4	3.3	1.6	2.9	2.3 (192)
Total	1.9 (317)	3.3 (299)	2.4 (117)	4.7 (116)	2.1 (65)	4.5 (86)	2.9 (1000)
* Level of significance	1%	N.S.	5%	1%	5%	5%	1%

manifested a similar trend. Thus among non-adopters fertility is lowest among the Hindus and still higher among the Christians and highest among the Muslims for the young and older cohorts except in the case of young Christians. Among those who have accepted temporary methods, surprisingly, fertility is more or less uniform the young and older cohorts of all the three communities. But for the sterilized persons it is significantly lower among the Hindus compared to the Christians and Muslims and not much difference is noticed between the latter two groups. Hence the demographic effectiveness of sterilization is very great among the Hindus and also among the young couples and not for the older cohorts. Thus the lower fertility of Hindus and younger cohorts in all the communities would have been influenced significantly by family planning per se.

Table 7.3 : Percentage of family planning adoption status according to different castes and religion

Caste groups	Number of Children ≤2	3+	Total
SC/ST	62.1 (58)	94.1 (79)	78.7 (137)
BC	66.7 (96)	92.1 (116)	78.5 (212)
Caste Hindus	72.3 (107)	92.0 (69)	79.0 (176)
Muslims	58.4 (38)	79.0 (69)	70.2 (106)
Fishermen Christians	31.1 (23)	61.7 (66)	50.8 (92)
Total	61.8* (322)	83.3* (399)	72.1* (1000)

* Level of a significant 1%.

Family Planning Adoption Status According to Religion and Caste

Religion and caste-wise variations in adoption of contraception are analysed in the present study. An overwhelming percentage (72%) of the total sample population have adopted one or the other methods of family planning. Among the three religious groups the level of adoption of contraception is lowest for the Fishermen Christians (50.8%) followed by the Muslims (70.2%), it is the highest among the Hindus (79%). When we control the number of children, an overwhelming proportion (83.3%) of couples with 3 and more number of children adopted family planning as against a significantly less number of couples with 2 and less number of children (61.8%). However, community wise differences are noticed in this adoption pattern. Another interesting observation is that among all the caste groups of the Hindus, there is not much variation in the proportion of adoption by the couple with three and more number of children, over 90 per cent of the scheduled castes, backward castes and the forward castes have adopted one or the other methods of contraception. But the rate of adoption of the couple with two and less number of children shows a direct relationship with the status of the caste groups. Among them more adopters are found in the forward castes (72%) followed by backward castes (66.7%) and lowest among the scheduled castes (62.1%). The difference in adoption between the forward castes and scheduled castes is statistically significant (significant at 1% level). It may be because of their differential socio-economic background and similarly, because of the differences in their infant and child mortality. A similar trend is noticed among the Muslims. But the rate of adoption by the low and high parity couples among the Muslims is lower than the scheduled caste and scheduled tribe among the Hindus. As expected the rate of adoption of contraception is lowest among the Fishermen Christians and very negligible (31.6%) among the families with two or less number of children. It is thus clear that the higher rate of fertility among the Fishermen Christians is because of very low level adoption of family planning methods. From these findings it is also confirmed that the adoption of family planning is a major determinant of fertility behaviour in Kerala among most of the communities, except people like the Fishermen Christians.

Education of Wife and Family Planning Adoption Status

Education shows a direct relationship with contraception at the aggregate level and also across the three religious groups. When the number of children is controlled the rate of adoption varies from 69.2 per cent to 100 and 48.2 to 77 per cent between illiterate and highly educated people with 3 and more children and ≤ 2 children respectively. Similar trend is noticed for the couples with three and more children irrespective of all the religious groups. But for couples with 2 children, a somewhat inconsistent trend is observed among the Hindus and Muslims. Among the Christians, however, a direct relationship is observed between education and adoption of contraception, irrespective of number of children.

When we consider the range of adoption of contraception on account of different educational status, it is much less among the Hindus (68 to 79% and 90 to 100%), a moderate increase observed among the Muslims (50 to 75% and 65 to 100%). An extensive difference is noticed among the Christians (25 to 75% and 55 to 94%). These findings indicate that the rate of adoption is significantly higher for the low and high parity couple among the Hindus followed by Muslims and Christians, which means that, other than education, the general differential development of these communities might be contributing to their differences in contraceptive acceptance. Further education level from class I to VII has much less impact in increasing the acceptance in contraception among the Hindus and young Christians but not older Christians and Muslims. However, when the education level increased to college level, the inter-community differences in contraception disappeared among all the three groups. Thus, higher education alone constitute the single most powerful factor to make all the communities accept family planning uniformly and in large proportions.

Table 7.4 : Percentage distribution of family planning adoption and education of wife according to religion and number of children

Education	Hindus		Christians		Muslims		Total	
	Number of children							
	≤2	3+	≤2	3+	≤2	3+	≤2	3+
Illiterates	67.9	90.3	25.0@	55.0	50.0@	65.0	48.2 (27)	69.2 (63)
1 - 4	68.6	90.9	30.8@	66.1	44.4@	71.4	54.7 (47)	77.0 (107)
5 - 7	65.8	92.0	30.0@	81.8	61.5@	83.3	61.6 (61)	89.0 (97)
8 - 10	64.8	93.1	56.7	94.1	60.0	95.5	63.0 (141)	93.7 (118)
College education	79.3	100.0	75.0@	-	75.0@	100.0	77.1 (27)	100.0 (14)
Total	68.2 (244)	92.2 (238)	40.8 (40)	68.9 (93)	58.5 (38)	79.1 (68)	61.8 (322)	83.3 (399)

Only adopters are given in the table.
@: Sample less than ten.

Family Planning Adoption Status and Income

According to the table 7.5, economic status of the family showed a positive association with the acceptance of contraception among couples with 2 or less children and 3 or more children in the population as a whole. However, the trend is more pronounced and the range of difference is greater among the couples with two or less children than three and more children. When we consider the same among the three communities, a similar trend is noticed across all the three groups among the couples with 2 and less children, but such a trend is not there among couples with 3 and more children for the Hindus and Christians. Of course, it is there, for the Muslims. Thus it is fairly confirmed here that income level of the family by and large is directly related to the acceptance of contraception. The absence of pronounced trend among the older couples might be because the differences in increase among them would not have been very large in the past as compared to at present.

Table 7.5 : Percentage distribution of family planning adoption status and family income according to religion and number of children

Income (in Rs.)	Hindus		Christians		Muslims		Total	
	Number of children							
	≤2	3+	≤2	3+	≤2	3+	≤2	3+
10,000	66.2	91.7	36.8	69.1	52.5	74.6	57.8 (192)	81.7 (268)
10,001-20,000	70.5	93.5	52.9	66.7	63.2	88.9	67.6 (100)	85.5 (112)
20,001+	72.4	92.3	60.0	100.0	83.3	100.0	73.2 (30)	95.0 (19)
Total	68.2 (244)	92.2 (238)	40.8 (40)	68.9 (93)	58.5 (38)	79.1 (68)	61.8 (322)	83.3 (399)

Note : Only adopters are given in the table.

Occupation and Family Planning Adoption Status

Occupational differences of the womenfolk and mobility are constitute certain differences in acceptance of family planning. In thc population as a whole, the single largest proportion of the women who are educated and employed in non-traditional avocations and the traditional labourers have adopted the largest proportions of contraceptives when they have two and less and three and more living children. But the differences in acceptance across the four occupational groups (Labourers, petty business, housewives and educated employee) is significant when they have two or less living children. Such a difference is not there when they achieved three and more living children. While examining occupational differences across the three religious groups no definite trend is noticed. However, among the Hindus, the rate of adoption is lower for the labourers and highest for the educated employees and almost an intermediate level for the women who employed in petty business and living as housewives in both the cases of low and high parity groups. But in the case of Muslims a more or less similar trend is noticed and in the Christians a reverse trend is noticed. Nevertheless, the proportion of adoption is more or less very high for the women who have moved to higher occupations among the Hindus and Muslims and such opportunity happens to be negligible among the Christians.

Table 7.6 : Percentage distribution of family planning adoption status and occupation of wife according to religion and number of children

Occupation of wife	Hindus		Christians		Muslims		Total	
	Number of children							
	≤2	3+	≤2	3+	≤2	3+	≤2	3+
Labourers	58.8	88.7	66.6	90.0	100.0	66.7	62.0 (44)	88.8 (71)
Petty business	75.0@	90.9	12.5@	68.7	100.0@	100.0	50.0 (9)	81.3 (26)
Housewives	69.4	92.7	37.5	64.2	53.6	78.1	61.6 (252)	82.2 (296)
Educated employees	72.2	100.0@	–	50.0@	80.0@	100.0	73.9 (17)	85.7 (6)
Total	68.2 (244)	92.2 (238)	40.8 (40)	68.9 (93)	58.5 (38)	79.1 (68)	61.8 (322)	83.3 (399)

Note : Only adopters are given in the table. @Sample less than ten.

Belief on Child Birth

A hypothesis that was considered here is that the belief of the couple about conception and child birth may have a bearing on acceptance of family planning. When the couple believe that child birth is an exclusive function of God, they are unlikely to accept contraception easily and in large numbers as against those who believe otherwise. When this cultural variable was correlated with acceptance of contraception the hypothesis is partially confirmed and also among the couple with three and more children in the population as a whole. The same trend is noticed among the Hindus, Christians and the Muslims for the similar cohorts of women. But it does not hold good for the cohorts of women with two or less children in all the communities. Hence the findings revealed that older women adopters alone may be subscribing to this concept and not the young women.

Table 7.7 : Percentage distribution of family planning adoption status and belief on child birth, religion and number of children

Children are blessings of God	Hindus		Christians		Muslims		Total	
	Number of Children							
	≤2	3+	≤2	3+	≤2	3+	≤2	3+
Yes	71.3	90.1	40.0	64.4	59.3	77.3	62.0 (199)	78.6 (268)
No	68.1	95.3	43.5	95.0	54.5	90.9	61.5 (123)	94.9 (131)
Total	68.2 (244)	92.3 (238)	40.8 (40)	68.9 (93)	58.5 (38)	79.1 (68)	61.8 (322)	83.3 (399)

Monetary Incentives

There are different forms of incentives now in vogue in the national family planning programme. It varies from state to state and also in different private and government organizations. Kerala, in particular, experimented with different types of incentives which included cash for the clients, and the motivators/change agents. It also included non-monetary incentives of different kinds. The famous Ernakulam camps held in 1973-1974 gave the maximum variety of incentives in the Indian family planning programme. An evaluation study conducted on this camp confirmed that nearly 50 per cent of the people adopted sterilization for the sake of incentives. In the light of the importance already experienced if incentives for motivating couples to accept family planning in Kerala, this factor forms yet another determinant of contraceptive behaviour.

Table 7.8 : Percentage distribution of family planning adoption and incentives status according to religion and number of children

Incentives	Hindus		Christians		Muslims		Total	
	Number of children							
	≤2	3+	≤2	3+	≤2	3+	2	3+
Not important	61.4	84.3	31.7	44.4	47.5	65.9	54.1 (132)	71.0 (120)
Important	73.8	96.4	47.4	77.7	76.0	92.9	68.6 (190)	90.0 (279)
Total	68.2 (244)	92.2 (238)	40.8 (40)	68.9 (93)	58.5 (38)	79.1 (68)	61.8 (322)	83.3 (399)

The table 7.8 confirmed the hypothesis that significantly more proportion of couples adopted family planning with two or less and three and more children, when they agreed with the importance of incentives in the population as a whole. The same trend is uniformly seen among the Hindus, Christians and Muslims with different number of living children. However, the range of difference in acceptance of family planning for the people who agreed or did not agreed with the incentives ranged from 12 per cent among the Hindus to 28 per cent among the Muslims and that of 33 per cent for the Christians. Hence, it is clear that the incentives played a relatively more important role among the Muslims and Christians than among the Hindus. Thus it is beyond any doubt that monetary incentives have a differential influence among different communities based on their socio-economic status and it is a crucial factor among the economically backward communities like Fishermen and Muslims for increased acceptance of family planning.

Table 7.9 : Percentage distribution of Family Planning adoption Status and number of male living Chidlren according to Religion and number of living children.

Number of male living children	Hindus		Christians		Muslims		Total	
	Number of Children							
	≤2	3+	≤2	3+	≤2	3+	≤2	3+
No male living children	60.7	96.8	28.6	58.3	61.9	-	54.2 (91)	82.6 (38)
1 child	66.1	93.3	47.4	67.7	54.5	82.4	61.7 (164)	84.9 (107)
2+ children	89.0	90.7	44.4	70.8	63.6	80.6	76.8 (67)	82.7 (254)
Total	68.2 (244)	92.2 (238)	40.8 (40)	68.9 (93)	58.5 (38)	79.1 (68)	61.8 (322)	83.3 (399)

Value of Son

Value of son is a composite variable which is endowed with an interdisciplinary influence viz., cultural, psychological, economic and social. These dimensions of value of children and their importance in regulating fertility behaviour is well established through the cross-cultural-cum-national studies conducted in several South-East Asian countries by the East West Population Institute (Arnold et al., 1977). Though it is very important as a determinant of fertility it is equally important to the determinant of family planning. Its pronatalist influence already been confirmed under the chapter on value of children and fertility behaviour. The two recent studies conducted in Kerala at micro and macro level also confirmed its pronatalist influence (Mahadevan and Sumangala, 1986; Mahadevan, 1986). In the light of this evidence it is hypothesised here that value of children acts as a major barrier for acceptance of family planning.

The table 7.9 partially confirmed the above hypothesis. It is true for the couples with two or less children but did not manifest similar trend for the couples with three and more children in the population as a whole. Number of male living children is directly related to the acceptance of contraception with all the couples with two or less living children. The same trend is observed across the three communities also with two and less children. However, with three and more children, a similar trend is noticed among the Christians alone and a reverse trend is noticed among the Hindus and Muslims. Thus the findings to a certain extent support the importance of value of children as a barrier for family planning. In most of the cases, adoption reached the peak period with two and more children. It may be because two sons are needed to avoid the risk involved in the possibility of childhood mortality which again may increase the risk in old age security. Therefore, certain social security measures may have to be introduced to minimise the adverse influence of value of children against the promotion of family planning programmes. It is interesting to note as an exceptional case, that the largest proportion of the Hindus adopted family planning with three and more children in the absence of a male child (97%) and also with one child (93%).

Induced Abortion

In the light of the Medical Termination of Pregnancy (MTP) act passed in India 1972, it was assumed that induced abortion would have increased as a method of fertility control in this population. However, it is not found to be true. Only 5.1 per cent of the total population resorted to induced abortion for the control of their fertility or for other reasons. The percentage varied between the Fishermen Christians (2.6%) on the one hand, and the Hindus (6.0%) and Muslims (5.3%) on the other hand. These figures indicate that only very few Christians followed this method to regulate their fertility, and more Hindus adopted it than others. Hence religious objection might be a factor for the Christians avoiding this method.

When the influence of abortion on fertility behaviour was examined for a population as a whole, it has not reduced the fertility (3.3 children) compared to others who have not adopted induced abortion (2.9). A similar trend is noticed among most of the communities and also across different age cohorts. Thus it may be probable that most women adopted induced abortion only after achieving the desired family size and also getting a large number of children. Thus it did not influence to regulate fertility. Its influence may be to avoid certain number of unwanted children.

Table 7.10 : Percentage distribution of respondents according to abortion and the three religious groups

Induced abortion	Hindus	Christians	Muslims	Total
No	94.0	97.4	94.7	94.9 (949)
Yes	6.0	2.6	5.3	5.1 (51)
Total	100.0 (616)	100.0 (233)	100.0 (151)	100.0 (1000)

EIGHT

PATH ANALYSIS

In this chapter the findings of a path analysis is presented. Out of the several multivariate analysis techniques, path analysis is considered in order to identify the direct, indirect and the individual influence of various independent variables on the dependent variable, fertility. Since, religion is controlled throughout the analysis, separate path analysis has been carried out for the Hindus, Christians and Muslims, besides carrying out a common analysis for the population as a whole. The major independent variables considered for this analysis include: Education, Opportunity cost, Value of children, Age at marriage, Breastfeeding, Family planning and lastly Fertility. In the path model also major proximate variables have been retained besides including the important sociological and other major determinants of fertility behaviour. The selection of the variables for the path analysis has been made, after examining their importance in the preceding tabulations. Nevertheless, only one proximate variable breastfeeding, which did not emerge as a major factor in the tabulations, is included here because it is an important proximate variable.

Path Analysis Technique

The main principle of path analysis is that any correlation coefficient between two variables, or overall measure of empirical relationship can be decomposed into a series of paths. Path analysis is a standardised multiple regression technique in which a chain of relationship among the variables arranged in an orderly manner, is examined through a series of regression analysis. Each dependent variable in this analysis is regarded as determined by the variables preceding it is in the path diagram. It is assumed that the set of variables considered in the path analysis is linearly additive and a symmetrical relationship exists among the variables.

Path Model for Fertility Data

According to the conceptualization of path diagram in figure 1, education of wife is considered as the most basic and comprehensive independent variable, which influence fertility behaviour directly and indirectly through most of the other independent variables. The other independent variables considered in the scheme of analysis are: Opportunity cost, value of children, Age at marriage of wife, Breastfeeding and Family Planning. All these variables have been ordered in the scheme of analysis on the basis of their logical position in influencing both directly and indirectly on fertility behaviour.

For analysing and assessing the influence of the preceding list of variables among the three religious groups and also for the population as a whole, similar attempts of analysis have been made in order to identify the differential influence of the path coefficient. It is assumed that all the independent variables considered here may have direct influence on fertility behaviour and some of them may also have indirect influence through other variables on fertility. The rank order of the influence of these variables may also be different among the three cultural groups. The path diagram in figure 1 has shown, the causal direction of the variables influencing fertility. Even though there are many paths through the independent variable, reaching the dependent variable (fertility) a few paths have been selected for calculating the indirect effect. It is done because such variables will have major and meaningful influence on fertility than considering all the variables for the same purpose.

The structural equations used for the analysis derived from the path diagrams are given below:

1. $X_0 = P_0X_1 + P_0X_2 + P_0X_3 + P_0X_4 + P_0X_5 + P_0X_6$

2. $X_6 = P_6X_1 + P_6X_2 + P_6X_3 + P_6X_4 + P_6X_5$

3. $X_4 = P_4X_1 + P_4X_2 + P_4X_3$

4. $X_3 = P_3X_1 + P_3X_2$

5. $X_5 = P_5X_1 + P_5X_2$

DIAGRAM

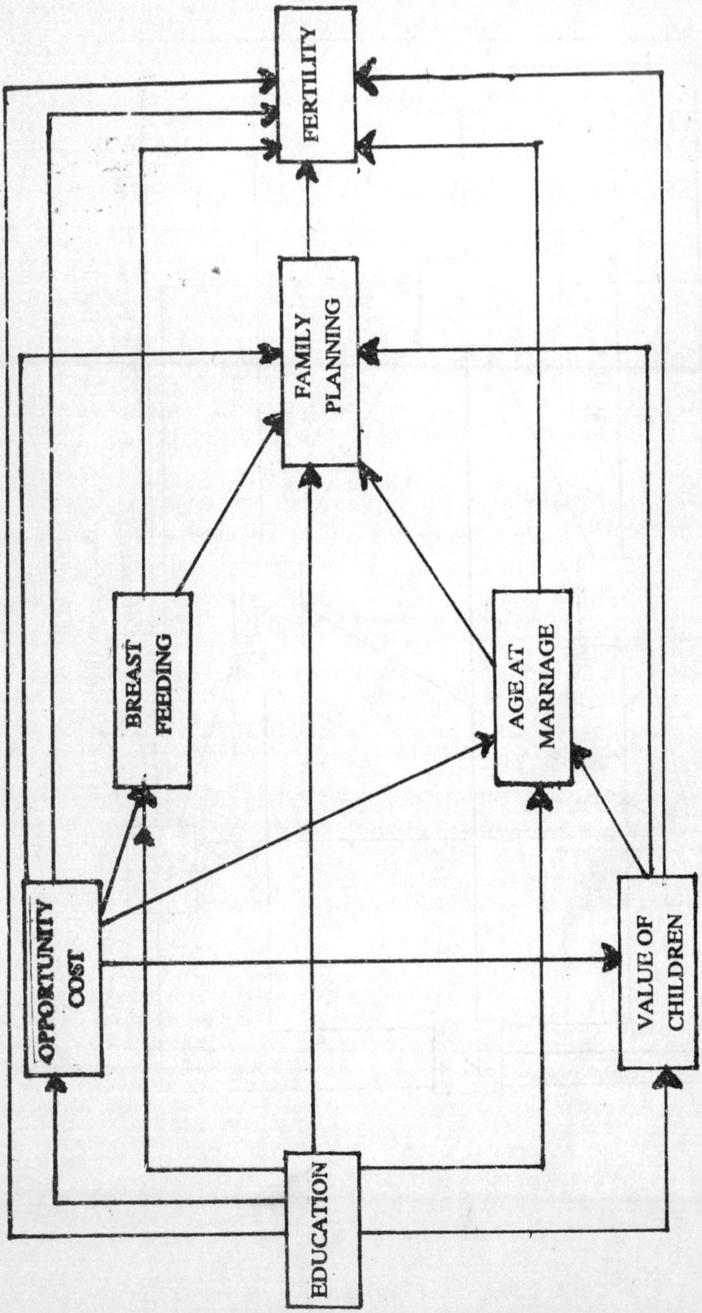
FERTILITY
FAMILY PLANNING
BREAST FEEDING
AGE AT MARRIAGE
OPPORTUNITY COST
VALUE OF CHILDREN
EDUCATION

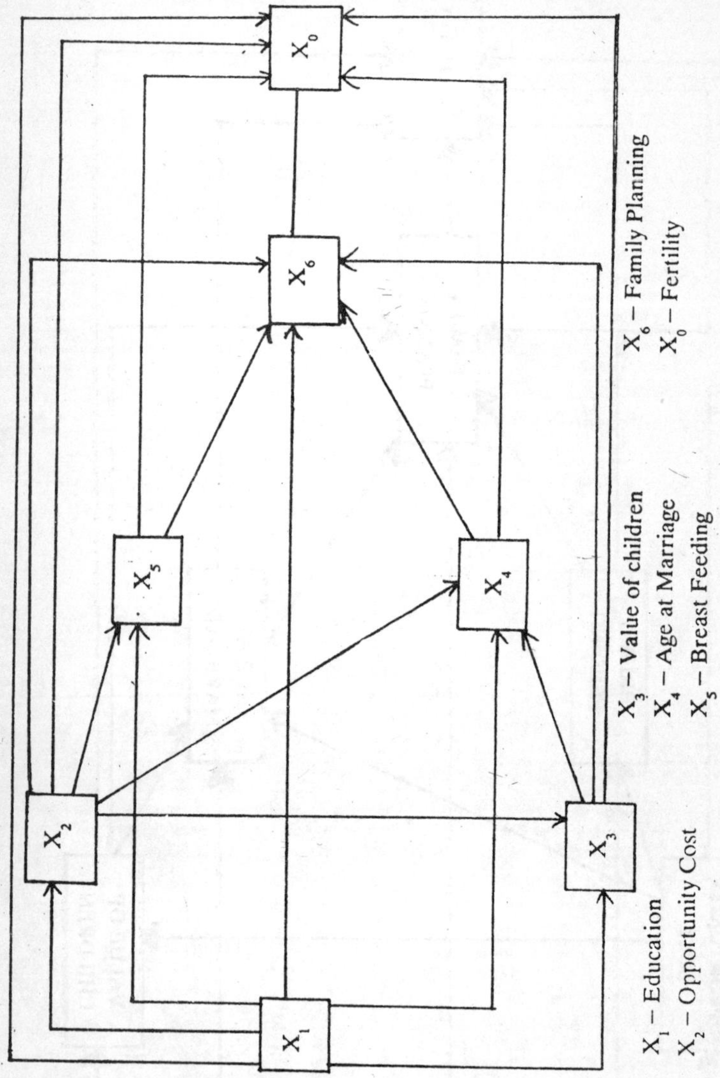
X_0
X_6
X_5
X_4
X_2
X_3
X_1
X_1 – Education
X_2 – Opportunity Cost
X_3 – Value of children
X_4 – Age at Marriage
X_5 – Breast Feeding
X_6 – Family Planning
X_0 – Fertility

Table 8.1 (a) Path Co-efficients for Fertility - Hindus

Path Co-efficient	Value
$P_{0,1}$	-0.162926
$P_{0,2}$	-0.381929
$P_{0,3}$	0.279068
$P_{0,4}$	-0.219647
$P_{0,5}$	0.497794
$P_{0,6}$	-0.307013
$P_{6,1}$	0.231717
$P_{6,2}$	0.076339
$P_{6,3}$	-0.615379
$P_{6,4}$	-0.014643
$P_{6,5}$	0.124477
$P_{4,1}$	0.150940
$P_{4,2}$	0.010989
$P_{4,3}$	0.085454
$P_{3,1}$	-0.211015
$P_{3,2}$	-0.173133
$P_{5,1}$	0.155926
$P_{5,2}$	0.187669

Path Diagram with Path Coefficient for fertility — HINDUS

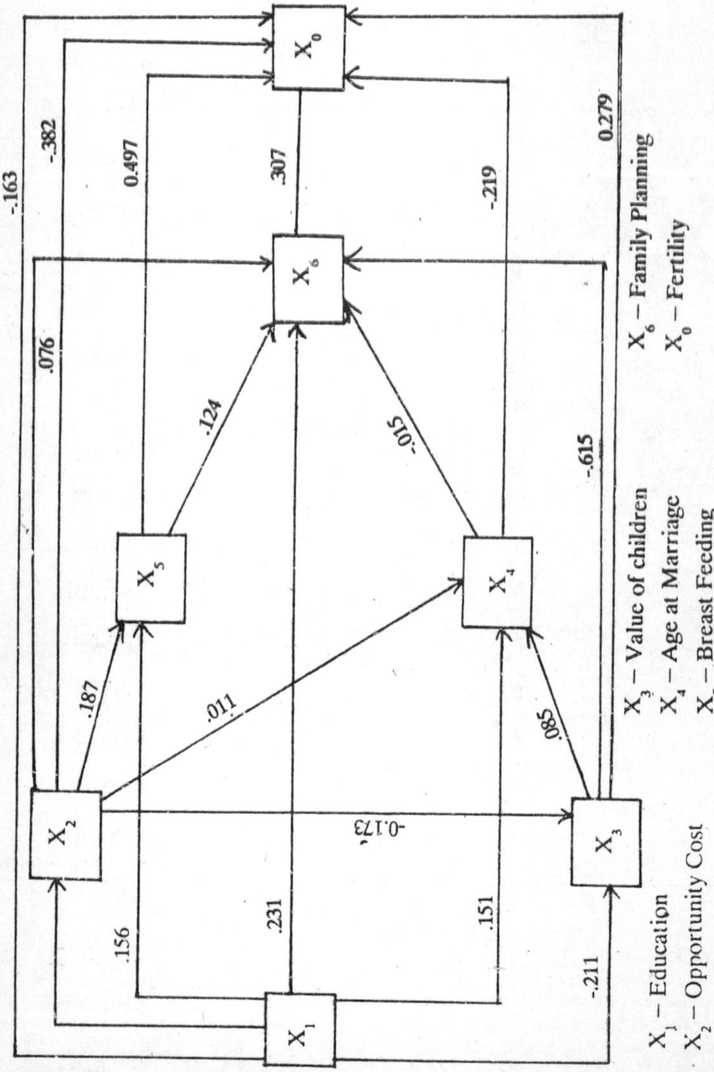

Table 8.1 (b) : Path Co-efficient for Fertility-Christians

Path Co-efficient	Value
$P_{0,1}$	-0.220863
$P_{0,2}$	-0.480977
$P_{0,3}$	0.201316
$P_{0,4}$	-0.299816
$P_{0,5}$	0.6553714
$P_{0,6}$	-0.019943
$P_{6,1}$	0.367291
$P_{6,2}$	-0.176905
$P_{6,3}$	0.044545
$P_{6,4}$	-0.182327
$P_{6,5}$	0.133660
$P_{4,1}$	0.418789
$P_{4,2}$	-0.0273030
$P_{4,3}$	-0.0305408
$P_{3,1}$	0.026408
$P_{3,2}$	-0.262494
$P_{5,1}$	0.161372
$P_{5,2}$	0.214749

Path Diagram with Path Coefficient for fertility — CHRISTIANS

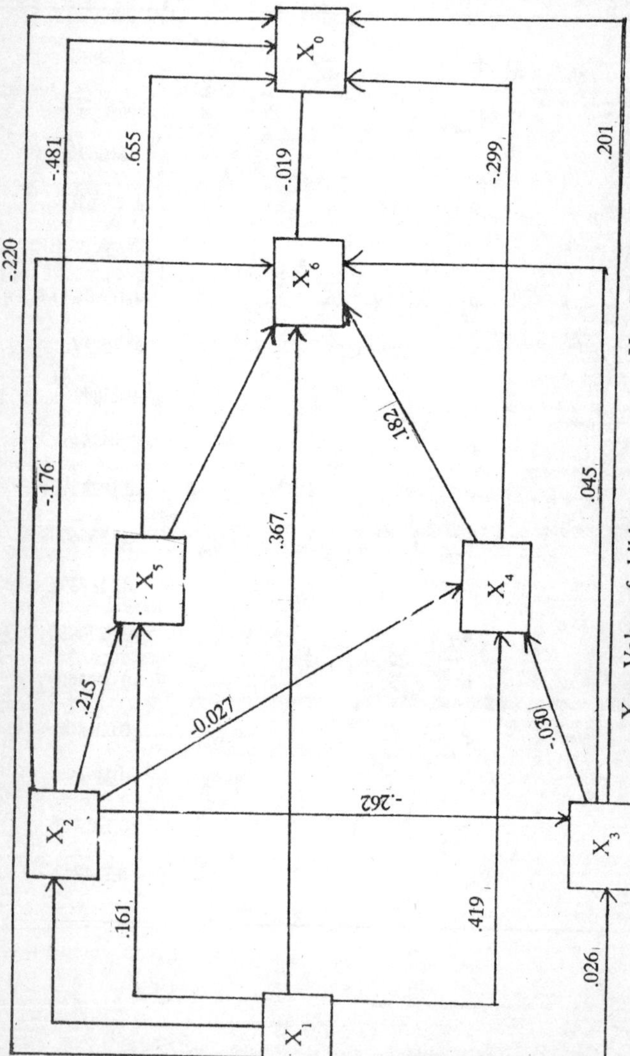

X_1 – Education
X_2 – Opportunity Cost
X_3 – Value of children
X_4 – Age at Marriage
X_5 – Breast Feeding
X_6 – Family Planning
X_0 – Fertility

Table 8.1 (c): Path Co-efficients for Fertility - Muslims

Path Co-efficient	Value
$P_{0,1}$	-0.168869
$P_{0,2}$	-0.458307
$P_{0,3}$	0.202419
$P_{0,4}$	-0.249725
$P_{0,5}$	0.468179
$P_{0,6}$	-0.153997
$P_{6,1}$	0.177009
$P_{6,2}$	-0.088088
$P_{6,3}$	-0.027198
$P_{6,4}$	0.111998
$P_{6,5}$	0.106060
$P_{4,1}$	0.341428
$P_{4,2}$	0.016920
$P_{4,3}$	0.113675
$P_{3,1}$	0.032244
$P_{3,2}$	-0.355587
$P_{5,1}$	0.248688
$P_{5,2}$	0.082563

Path Diagram with Path Coefficient for fertility — MUSLIMS

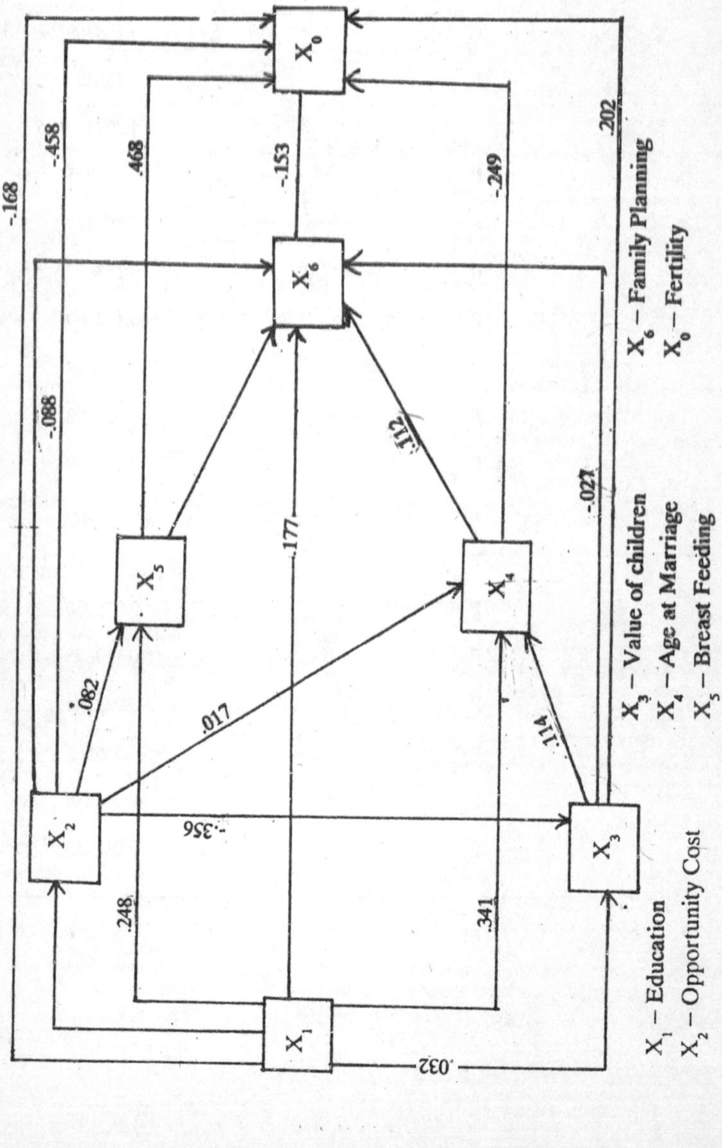

Table 8.1 (d) : Path Co-efficients for Fertility (Total Population)

Path Co-efficient	Value
$P_{0,1}$	-0.225425
$P_{0,2}$	-0.367779
$P_{0,3}$	0.202362
$P_{0,4}$	-0.244091
$P_{0,5}$	0.213259
$P_{0,6}$	-0.161258
$P_{6,1}$	0.201239
$P_{6,2}$	-0.037404
$P_{6,3}$	-0.063205
$P_{6,4}$	-0.032109
$P_{6,5}$	0.105475
$P_{4,1}$	0.251804
$P_{4,2}$	0.040908
$P_{4,3}$	0.053768
$P_{3,1}$	-0.048866
$P_{3,2}$	-0.022076
$P_{5,1}$	0.165802
$P_{5,2}$	0.176101

Path Diagram with Path Coefficient for fertility — TOTAL POPULATION

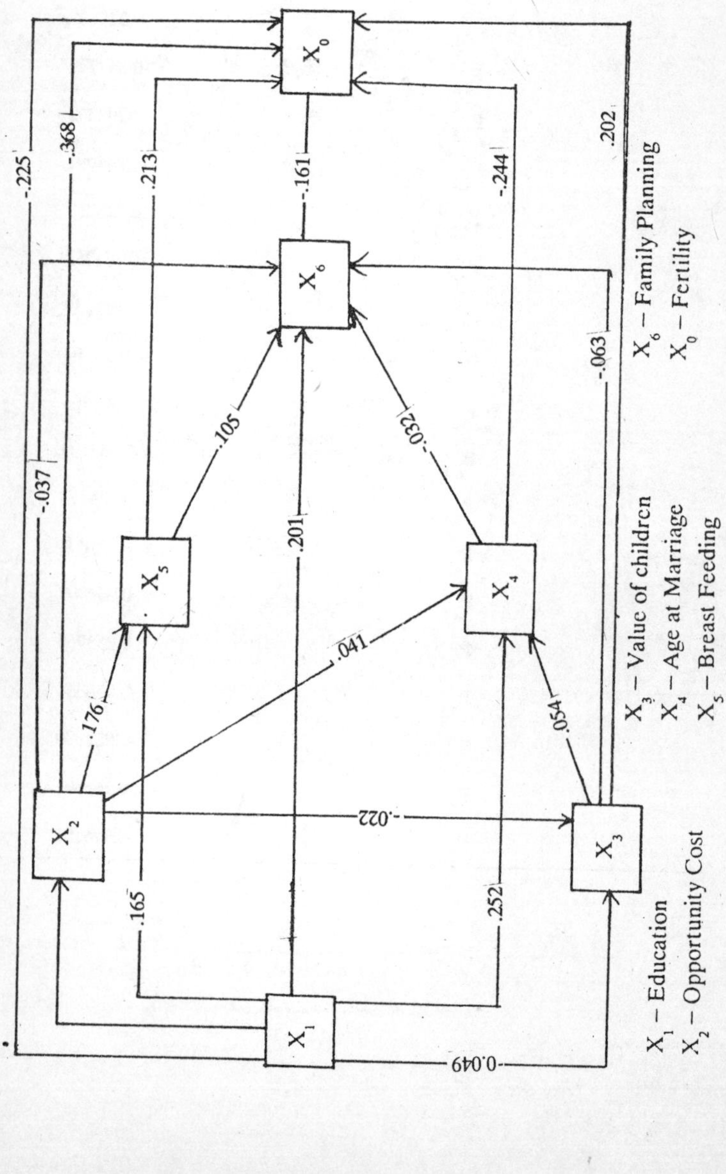

Table 8.2 (a): Direct and Indirect effects of the variables as per the path diagram for Fertility - Hindus

Equation	Path-Co-efficient	Value
	Direct Effects	
$X_1 \quad X_0$	$P_{0,1}$	-0.162926
$X_2 \quad X_0$	$P_{0,2}$	-0.381929
$X_3 \quad X_0$	$P_{0,3}$	0.279068
$X_4 \quad X_0$	$P_{0,4}$	-0.219647
$X_5 \quad X_0$	$P_{0,5}$	0.497794
$X_6 \quad X_0$	$P_{0,6}$	-0.307013
	Indirect Effects	
$X_1 \quad X_3 \quad X_0$	$P_{3,1} \, P_{0,3}$	-0.058880
$X_1 \quad X_3 \quad X_4 \quad X_0$	$P_{3,1} \, P_{4,3} \, P_{0,4}$	0.003960
$X_1 \quad X_3 \quad X_4 \quad X_6 \quad X_0$	$P_{3,1} \, P_{4,3} \, P_{6,4} \, P_{0,6}$	-0.000081
$X_1 \quad X_4 \quad X_0$	$P_{4,1} \, P_{0,4}$	-0.033153
$X_1 \quad X_4 \quad X_6 \quad X_0$	$P_{4,1} \, P_{6,4} \, P_{0,6}$	0.000678
$X_1 \quad X_5 \quad X_0$	$P_{5,1} \, P_{0,5}$	0.077620
$X_1 \quad X_5 \quad X_6 \quad X_0$	$P_{5,1} \, P_{6,5} \, P_{0,6}$	-0.005959
$X_1 \quad X_6 \quad X_0$	$P_{6,1} \, P_{0,6}$	-0.071137
$X_2 \quad X_3 \quad X_0$	$P_{3,2} \, P_{0,3}$	-0.048314
$X_2 \quad X_3 \quad X_4 \quad X_0$	$P_{3,2} \, P_{4,3} \, P_{0,4}$	0.003249
$X_2 \quad X_3 \quad X_4 \quad X_6 \quad X_0$	$P_{3,2} \, P_{4,3} \, P_{6,4} \, P_{0,6}$	-0.000066
$X_2 \quad X_4 \quad X_0$	$P_{4,2} \, P_{0,4}$	-0.002413
$X_2 \quad X_4 \quad X_6 \quad X_0$	$P_{4,2} \, P_{6,4} \, P_{0,6}$	0.000049
$X_2 \quad X_5 \quad X_0$	$P_{5.2} \, P_{0,5}$	-0.093420
$X_2 \quad X_5 \quad X_6 \quad X_0$	$P_{5,2} \, P_{6,5} \, P_{0,6}$	-0.007172
$X_2 \quad X_6 \quad X_0$	$P_{6,2} \, P_{0,6}$	-0.023437

X_3 X_4 X_0	$P_{4,3}$ $P_{0,4}$	-0.018769
X_3 X_4 X_6 X_0	$P_{4,3}$ $P_{6,4}$ $P_{0,6}$	0.000384
X_4 X_6 X_0	$P_{6,4}$ $P_{0,6}$	0.004494
X_5 X_6 X_0	$P_{6,5}$ $P_{0,6}$	-0.038210

Table 8.2 (b) : Direct and Indirect Effects of the Variables as per the path diagram for Fertility - Christians

Equation	Path Co-efficient	Value
	<u>Direct effect</u>	
X_1 X_0	$P_{0,1}$	-0.220863
X_2 X_0	$P_{0,2}$	-0.480977
X_3 X_0	$P_{0,3}$	0.201316
X_4 X_0	$P_{0,4}$	-0.299816
X_5 X_0	$P_{0,5}$	0.6553714
X_6 X_0	$P_{0,6}$	-0.019943
	<u>Indirect effect</u>	
X_1 X_3 X_0	$P_{3,1}$ $P_{0,3}$	0.005314
X_1 X_3 X_4 X_0	$P_{3,1}$ $P_{4,3}$ $P_{0,4}$	0.000242
X_1 x_3 X_4 X_6 X_0	$P_{3,1}$ $P_{4,3}$ $P_{6,4}$ $P_{0,6}$	-0.000003
X_1 X_4 X_0	$P_{4,1}$ $P_{0,4}$	-0.125557
X_1 X_4 X_6 X_0	$P_{4,1}$ $P_{6,4}$ $P_{0,6}$	0.001520
X_1 X_5 X_0	$P_{5,1}$ $P_{0,5}$	0.105757
X_1 X_5 X_6 X_0	$P_{5,1}$ $P_{6,5}$ $P_{0,6}$	-0.002108
X_1 X_6 X_0	$P_{6,1}$ $P_{0,6}$	-0.007323
X_2 X_3 X_0	$P_{3,2}$ $P_{0,3}$	-0.052840
X_2 X_3 X_4 X_0	$P_{3,2}$ $P_{4,3}$ $P_{0,4}$	-0.002403
X_2 X_3 X_4 X_6 X_0	$P_{3.2}$ $P_{4,3}$ $P_{6,4}$ $P_{0,6}$	0.000029

X_2 X_4 X_0	$P_{4,2}$ $P_{0,4}$	0.008185
X_2 X_4 X_6 X_0	$P_{4,2}$ $P_{6,4}$ $P_{0,6}$	-0.000099
X_2 X_5 X_0	$P_{5,2}$ $P_{0,5}$	0.140734
X_2 X_5 X_6 X_0	$P_{5,2}$ $P_{6,5}$ $P_{0,6}$	-0.000572
X_2 X_6 X_0	$P_{6,2}$ $P_{0,6}$	0.003527
X_3 X_4 X_6	$P_{4,3}$ $P_{0,4}$	0.009156
X_3 X_4 X_6 X_0	$P_{4,3}$ $P_{6,4}$ $P_{0,6}$	-0.000111
X_4 X_6 X_0	$P_{6,4}$ $P_{0,6}$	0.003635
X_5 X_6 X_0	$P_{6,5}$ $P_{0,6}$	-0.002665

Table 8.2 (c): Direct and indirect effect of the variables as per the path diagram for Fertility - Muslims

Equation	Path Co-efficent	Value
	Direct effect	
X_1 X_0	$P_{0,1}$	-0.168869
X_2 X_0	$P_{0,2}$	-0.458307
X_3 X_0	$P_{0,3}$	0.202419
X_4 X_0	$P_{0,4}$	-0.249725
X_5 X_0	$P_{0,5}$	0.468179
X_6 X_0	$P_{0,6}$	-0.153997
	Indirect effect	
X_1 X_3 X_0	$P_{3,1}$ $P_{0,3}$	0.006526
X_1 X_3 X_4 X_0	$P_{3,1}$ $P_{4,3}$ $P_{0,4}$	-0.000915
X_1 X_3 X_4 X_6 X_0	$P_{3,1}$ $P_{4,3}$ $P_{6,4}$ $P_{0,6}$	-0.000063
X_1 X_4 X_0	$P_{4,1}$ $P_{0,4}$	-0.085262
X_1 X_4 X_6 X_0	$P_{4,1}$ $P_{6,4}$ $P_{0,6}$	-0.005888

X_1 X_5 X_0	$P_{5,1}$ $P_{0,5}$	0.116427
X_1 X_5 X_6 X_0	$P_{5,1}$ $P_{6,5}$ $P_{0,6}$	-0.004059
X_1 X_6 X_0	$P_{6,1}$ $P_{0,6}$	-0.027256
X_2 X_3 X_0	$P_{3,2}$ $P_{0,3}$	-0.071977
X_2 X_3 X_4 X_0	$P_{3,2}$ $P_{4,3}$ $P_{0,4}$	0.010094
X_2 X_3 X_4 X_6 X_0	$P_{3,2}$ $P_{4,3}$ $P_{6,4}$ $P_{0,6}$	0.000697
X_2 X_4 X_0	$P_{4,2}$ $P_{0,4}$	-0.004225
X_2 X_4 X_6 X_0	$P_{4,2}$ $P_{6,4}$ $P_{0,6}$	-0.000292
X_2 X_5 X_0	$P_{5,2}$ $P_{0,5}$	0.038652
X_2 X_5 X_6 X_0	$P_{5,2}$ $P_{6,5}$ $P_{0,6}$	-0.001347
X_2 X_6 X_0	$P_{6,2}$ $P_{0,6}$	0.013565
X_3 P_4 X_0	$P_{4,3}$ $P_{0,4}$	-0.028385
X_3 X_4 X_6 X_0	$P_{4,3}$ $P_{6,4}$ $P_{0,6}$	-0.001960
X_4 X_6 X_0	$P_{6,4}$ $P_{0,6}$	-0.017245
X_5 X_6 X_0	$P_{6,5}$ $P_{0,6}$	-0.016324

Table 8.2 (d): Direct and Indirect effects of the variables as per the path diagram for fertility - Total population

Equation Value		Path Co-efficient
	<u>Direct effect</u>	
X_1 X_0	$P_{0,1}$	-0.225425
X_2 X_0	$P_{0,2}$	-0.367779
X_3 X_0	$P_{0,3}$	0.202362
X_4 X_0	$P_{0,4}$	-0.244091
X_5 X_0	$P_{0,5}$	0.213259
X_6 X_0	$P_{0,6}$	-0.161258

Indirect effect		
$X_1\ X_3\ X_0$	$P_{3,1}\ P_{0,3}$	-0.009888
$X_1\ X_3\ X_4\ X_0$	$P_{3,1}\ P_{4,3}\ P_{0,4}$	0.000642
$X_1\ X_3\ X_4\ X_6\ X_0$	$P_{3,1}\ P_{4,3}\ P_{6,4}\ P_{0,6}$	-0.000014
$X_1\ X_4\ X_0$	$P_{4,1}\ P_{0,4}$	-0.061463
$X_1\ X_4\ X_6\ X_0$	$P_{4,1}\ P_{6,4}\ P_{0,6}$	0.001303
$X_1\ X_5\ X_0$	$P_{5,1}\ P_{0,5}$	0.035358
$X_1\ X_5\ X_6\ X_0$	$P_{5,1}\ P_{6,5}\ P_{0,6}$	-0.002813
$X_2\ X_6\ X_0$	$P_{6,1}\ P_{0,6}$	-0.032451
$X_2\ X_3\ X_0$	$P_{3,2}\ P_{0,3}$	0.0044673
$X_2\ X_3\ X_4\ X_0$	$P_{3,2}\ P_{4,3}\ P_{0,4}$	0.000289
$X_2\ X_3\ X_4\ X_6\ X_0$	$P_{3,2}\ P_{4,3}\ P_{6,4}\ P_{0,6}$	-0.000061
$X_2\ X_4\ X_0$	$P_{4,2}\ P_{0,4}$	-0.009985
$X_2\ X_4\ X_6\ X_0$	$P_{4,2}\ P_{6,4}\ P_{0,6}$	0.000212
$X_2\ X_5\ X_0$	$P_{5,2}\ P_{0,5}$	0.037555
$X_2\ X_5\ X_6\ X_0$	$P_{5,2}\ P_{6,5}\ P_{0,6}$	-0.002995
$X_2\ X_6\ X_0$	$P_{6,2}\ P_{0,6}$	0.006032
$X_3\ X_4\ X_0$	$P_{4,3}\ P_{0,4}$	-0.013124
$X_3\ X_4\ X_6\ X_0$	$P_{4,3}\ P_{6,4}\ P_{0,6}$	0.000278
$X_4\ X_6\ X_0$	$P_{6,4}\ P_{0,6}$	0.005177
$X_5\ X_6\ X_0$	$P_{6,5}\ P_{0,6}$	-0.017009

Table 8.3 (a): Direct, Indirect and Total effects of six variables on fertility - Hindus

Variable	Direct	Indirect	Total
Education (X_1)	-0.162926	-0.086952	-0.249878
Opportunity cost (X_2)	-0.381929	0.015316	-0.366613
Value of children (X_3)	0.279068	-0.018385	0.260683
Age at marriage (X_4)	-0.219647	0.004494	-0.215153
Breastfeeding (X_5)	0.497794	-0.038216	0.459578
Family planning (X_6)	-0.307013	-	-0.307013

Table 8.3 (b) : Direct, Indirect and Total effect of six variables on fertility - Christians

Variables	Direct	Indirect	Total
Education (X_1)	-0.220863	-0.0221575	-0.2430205
Opportunity cost (X_2)	-0.480977	0.0030325	-0.477952
Value of children (X_3)	0.201316	0.009046	0.210361
Age at marriage (X_4)	-0.299816	0.003635	-0.296181
Breastfeeding (X_5)	0.655371	-0.002665	0.652706
Family Planning (X_6)	-0.019943	—	-0.019943

Table 8.3 (c): Direct, Indirect and Total effects of six variables on fertility - Muslims

Variable	Direct	Indirect	Total
Education (X_1)	-0.168869	-0.00049	-0.169359
Opportunity cost (X_2)	-0.458307	-0.014833	-0.47314
Value of children (X_3)	0.202419	-0.030345	0.172074
Age at marriage (X_4)	-0.249725	-0.017245	-0.26697
Breastfeeding (X_5)	0.468179	-0.016324	0.451855
Family Planning (X_6)	-0.153997	-	-0.153997

Table 8.3 (d): Direct, Indirect and Total effects of six variables on fertility - Total Population

Variable	Direct	Indirect	Total
Education (X_1)	-0.225425	-0.060326	-0.294751
Opportunity cost (X_2)	-0.367779	0.0265797	-0.341199
Value of children (X_3)	0.202362	-0.012846	0.18896
Age at marriage (X_4)	-0.244091	0.005177	-0.238914
Breastfeeding (X_5)	0.213259	-0.017009	0.19625
Family planning (X_6)	-0.161258	-	-0.161258

Table 8.4 : Total effects of each variable for Hindus, Christians, Muslims

Variable	Hindus	Christians	Muslims	Total
X_1 Education	-0.249878	-0.243020	-0.169359	-0.662257
X_2 Opportunity cost	-0.366613	-0.477952	-0.47314	-1.317705
X_3 Value of children	0.260683	0.210361	0.172074	0.643118
X_4 Age at marriage	-0.215153	-0.296181	-0.26697	0.778304
X_5 Breastfeeding	0.459578	0.652706	0.451855	1.564139
X_6 Family Planning	-0.307013	-0.019943	-0.153997	-0.480953

Table 8.5 : Path Analysis Result, Rank Order

Variable	Hindus	Christians	Muslims
Breastfeeding	2	1	3
Opportunity cost	3	1	2
Age at marriage	3	1	2
Education	1	2	3
Value of children	1	2	3
Family planning	1	3	2

Breastfeeding

The duration of breastfeeding has shown uniformly positive and significant pronatalist effect on fertility for the population as a whole and for the three communities. Among all the six variables considered here for path analysis, this is the only variable that has no definite antinatalist influence for the fertility reduction. For the total population, its value ranked only in the fifth position (0.19625). But for the communities it was placed as the first factor. Among them, its influence was ranked highest for the Christians (0.652706) followed by the Hindus (0.459578) and lowest among the Muslims (0.451855). The same trend was already reported in the earlier chapter on breastfeeding About its direct influence on fertility the Christians showed highest value (0.655371) followed by the Hindus (0.497794) and the Muslims (0.468179). But at the same time its indirect influence was lowest among the Christians (-0.002665) and also not significant for all the three communities (see table 8.3 a,b,c and d).

From these findings it is confirmed that the influence of breastfeeding on fertility reduction is very negligible. The reasons for this findings may be that most of the people, who have had long duration of breastfeeding would also have attained high fertility. On the other hand younger women may not be breastfeeding for a longer period and also may have lower fertility. However, further in-depth study focussing mostly on this theme is needed to make a definite conclusion on this factor.

Opportunity Cost

An index on opportunity cost, consisting of the factors like: no scope for getting rest; unable to enjoy leisure time; no time to read and acquire knowledge; inconvenience in taking treatment; paucity of time to look after all the children; inadequate opportunity for school and college education have been taken together for measuring its influence on fertility behaviour. Out of the six factors considered in the path analysis, it showed the highest influence on fertility reduction on the population as a whole (-0.34119) and also among the three communities. However, its influence was ranked for the highest among the Christians (-0.477952) followed by the Muslims (-0.47314) and lowest among the Hindus (-0.366613). It was highly significant (1% level) for the total population and all the three communities. It has also shown a very high direct influence in all the three communities. But in their order of importance it is high among the Christians (-0.480977), followed by the Muslims (-0.458307) and the Hindus (-0.381929). Regarding its indirect influence, it is not significant among all the communities.

In view of its high importance in influencing fertility behaviour directly, highest priority may be given to manipulate its influence in controlling the fertility. Therefore, necessary health education and population education, on salient aspects of opportunity cost may be imparted among the eligible couples for controlling their fertility.

Age at Marriage

Age at marriage of wife manifests a significant inverse relationship with fertility behaviour uniformly for the population as a whole and the three religious groups. For the total population, its influence ranked next to education and occupies a third place (-0.238914) for the fertility reducing factors. Its relationship is significant at 5% level with fertility. Among the three communities it showed second place among all the variables and showed significant influence on fertility, next only to the opportunity cost. Regarding its influence among the three religious groups it also ranked first for the Christians (-0.296181) followed by the Muslims (-0.26697) and the Hindus (-0.215153). However, its influence is significant at 1% level for the Christians and Muslims and 5% level for the Hindus. It also showed direct and indirect effect on fertility behaviour. However, the direct effect is only significant for all the religious groups and the total population. For the population as a whole direct effect is significant at 1% level (-0.244091). Among the three religious groups its direct effect is significant at 1% level for the Christians (-0.299816) and Muslims (-0.249725), but for the Hindus it is at 5% level (-0.219647) (see table 8.3 a,b,c).

From these findings it is confirmed that the influence of age at marriage of women on fertility behaviour is differentially among the three communities and the direct influence is a common pattern of relationship. Hence measures should be introduced for the late marriage of women for controlling the fertility. It is highly advantageous for readucing fertility. Further, knowing the inadequate influence of this factor for certain communities notably among the Hindus may strengthen our efforts to increase their age at marriage.

Education

Education of the women also has shown a uniform negative association with fertility behaviour for the population as a whole and for the three communities. For the population as a whole it emerged as the second most important variable depressing the fertility behaviour (-0.294751). Its relationship is significant at 1% level with fertility. As regards its influence among the three communities, it is ranked first among the Hindus (-0.249878) followed by the Christians (-0.243020), and lastly among the Muslims (-0.19359). However, it showed third place among the variables that have negative association with fertility next only to age at marriage. It showed both direct and indirect influence on fertility behaviour, but the direct influence is more than the indirect. For the population as a whole direct influence is significant at 5% level and indirect influence is not statistically significant (see table 8.3 d).

Among the three communities, the direct influence of education is significant at 5% level for all of them. Regarding the direct effect of education it is greater for the Christians (-0.220863), followed by the Muslims (-0.168869) and the Hindus (-0.162926). On the other hand indirect effect of education is highest among the Hindus (-0.086952). Education being a key variable, which manifest both direct and indirect effect, may be given the highest priority for the control of fertility. Though Kerala's literacy rate is the highest among all the states in India, its influence on fertility reduction is considered as a model for the other low literacy states. Hence necessary steps may be taken for the improvement of education for the less educated group like Fishermen Christians and Muslims for controlling their high fertility.

Value of Children

The influence of value of children on fertility behaviour has shown in the lines of a positive association with fertility behaviour, that means greater the value attached to sons higher the fertility. For the population as a whole it has the fourth place (0.18896) and it is significant at 5% level. It has been differentially confirmed among the three cultural groups, while it is highly significant for the Hindus (1%) and is moderately significant among the Christians and

Muslims (5%). It showed more direct effect than the indirect effect. On the total population, its direct influence is (0.202362) significant at 5% level. Among the three communities, its direct influence is highest among the Hindus (0.279068) followed by the Muslims (0.20419) and the Christians (0.201316). But indirect effect is not significant.

Since this variable has mostly direct effect on fertility, highest priority should be given to minimize the pronatalist influence of this factor particularly among the Hindus. Hence differential strategy may have to be evolved to manipulate this variable among different religious groups.

Family Planning

Acceptance of family planning has been considered here as the sixth and last factor for this path analysis. As expected, it has proved to be a significant fertility regulating factor (sig. at 1% level) only among the Hindus. But not statistically significant among the Muslims and the Christians. In the order of its influence among the three communities, it is ranked as the first among the Hindus (-0.307013) followed by the Muslims (-0.153997) and lastly among the Christians (-0.019943). For the population as a whole also it is not statistically significant (-0.161258). It showed a negative association with fertility. It manifests only a direct relationship. Compared to the preceding factors of the determinants of fertility behaviour family planning emerged only as the sixth factor in the order of importance.

Thus, out of the six major factors of determinants of fertility behaviour studied here under path analysis viz., education, opportunity cost, value of children, age at marriage, breastfeeding and family planning. Only the first four factors alone were found to be very crucial and significant in regulating fertility behaviour. These factors have shown differential influence among the three cultural groups. The social (education), economic (opportunity cost), cultural (value of children) and proximate variables (age at marriage, breastfeeding and family planning) are important determinants of fertility behaviour on a differential basis across different cultural groups. Hence, the new population policy and family planning interventions may have to be consider these factors to modify, expand and improve the policy and programme strategy to control fertility on a scientific and expeditious basis in this part of our country.

NINE

SUMMARY AND IMPLICATIONS

The Problem and Method

The present study was undertaken to identify the influence of major demographic, developmental and socio-cultural determinants of differential fertility among the three religious groups, viz., the Hindus, Christians and Muslims in the Southern-most district of Kerala. Three religious groups were selected for the present study in view of the differential fertility prevailing among them. Of course, fertility studies started in Kerala as early as in 1960s, but they were mostly based on secondary data, census and sample registration schemes and also focussed on socio-economic and demographic variables (Kurup, 1963; Namboodiri, 1964; Nayar, 1982; Mahadevan, 1986 and 1987). Further, most of the earlier major studies separately did not cover all the religious groups, despite knowing their differential fertility. Hence, the present study is not only innovative but bridges the existing gap of knowledge on determinants of religious differentials in fertility. Added to this, it also specifically explains the direct and indirect influence of the crucial demographic, developmental and socio-cultural variables through the path analysis, which is now attempted for the first time in a Kerala population.

The location of the study was mainly in three community development blocks in Trivandrum district. This district was selected purposively because of its representative character with most of the other districts in Travancore region. The major objectives of the study were to examine the influence of each of the demographic variables, viz., Age at marriage, breastfeeding, contraception and birth interval besides important socio-economic and social change variables and value of children on fertility among the three major religious groups. This study also examined the differential fertility existing between the younger and older cohorts of women. One thousand eligible couples (women) were selected as respondents of the present research on the basis of a multi-stage random sampling procedure. Numerically, the Hindus constitute the largest segment of the population. Christians of the sample mostly belong to the Fishermen community because in Trivandrum district, other groups of Christians are negligible in the rural population. The universe of the study belongs to only rural areas. The data was collected by the Interview method using a detailed quasi-structured schedule. The analysis was carried out using computer facility. Religion and the duration of married life of wives were controlled throughout the analysis. In addition to the tabulations, "t" test was used for testing the level of significance; finally a path analysis was also used separately for all the three religious groups and the total population.

II Findings and Implications:

1. *Social Change and Differential Fertility*

During the last half a century period extensive social change on various aspects of society had taken place in Kerala on a differential basis among the three religious groups. As a result of social change, the Hindus in general have progressed, modernized and improved their quality of life considerably, but the Fishermen Christians and Muslims, though very much changed from their traditional setup, still lag behind when compared to the former. However, non-Fishermen Christians have progressed considerably in most aspects of life even when compared to the Hindus but they are not available in sufficient numbers in the study area and hence not covered in the present study. According to Rao (1957), even the Malabar region, which is the most backward region in the whole of Kerala, has undergone tremendous transformation in the field of occupation, family life, religious activities, leisure time activities and other various activities in the community in general. Similarly, according to Sreedhara Menon (1979), the 19th and 20th centuries witnessed the emergence of a new social order in Kerala under the impact of diverse social, economic and cultural influences. The British and Indian administrators, who were motivated by liberal impulses introduced in the early decades of the 19th century a series of administrative and social reforms with a view to modernizing administration and society in this state. As a result of all these governmental and voluntary efforts, several changes have taken place throughout

Kerala. Voluntary efforts were in fact, greater than the governmental efforts. Various religious and caste leaders and their organizations invested time, resources and energy for the modernization and development of their respective communities. The pioneering Social reform movements championed by the several leaders, viz., Chattampi Swamikal, Sri Narayana Guru, Mannath Padmanabhan, Ayyankali, Vakkom Abdul Khadar Moulvi, who belonged to different castes and religious groups in Kerala, helped to organise the religious communities on a competitive basis and on modern lines (Menon, 1979). They also liberated their fellowmen from outdated customs and life styles.

Chains of educational institutions, hospitals, periodicals, and papers were started on a competitive basis, which contributed to rapid social change among the people in general. In this context the pioneering efforts of the progressive and modern writers have to be emphasised for their inspiring contributions through dramas, novels, stories and poems in transforming the literary world and the people at large (Puthenkalam, 1977). The mass media also played a tremendous role in Kerala's social change. Kerala has the largest circulation of vernacular newspapers in India and also different types of vernacular periodicals. Their availability in remote areas was assured through the chain of thousands of libraries (4,977 in 1985) functioning all over the state which is a rare thing even in a developed country. Added to this, periodic changes and reforms introduced by different governments, with varied political philosophy, also worked on competitive basis for the welfare of the poor people in particular. All the successive governments gave the highest priority for education, health services, housing and many other social amenities of life. Parallelly the large scale migration of people from Kerala to urban areas within the state, within the country and to other countries, improved their economic status, life style and modernized their families in particular and villages in general (Mahadevan, 1987; Nair, 1983).

As a result of the individual, institutional, governmental and voluntary efforts, besides the natural influence of migration and mass media, Kerala has emerged as a modern state. The literacy rate of women in Kerala (64.5) is not only one of the highest in India, but can also be compared with many developed countries. Their occupational mobility within and outside Kerala is phenomenal. Kerala has the distinction of electing the largest proportion of women legislators, appointing the largest number of women teachers, health workers, lawyers, judges and other professionals, in India. The largest number of nurses working in India and abroad come from Kerala. Through all these new roles the status of women in Kerala has phenomenally improved though per capita income is still relatively low in Kerala (Rs. 677 in 1981-82) compared to other states in India. Most of the poor and middle class people have benefited from the government's poverty alleviation programmes. They have secured a house or house site, received an unemployment allowance or an old age pension and also some land through the land reforms. All this has contributed to the social and economic change for the vast majority of the middle class and poor people. Their health conditions are being well looked after by the state and voluntary agencies and they also extensively make use of the existing facilities. Over 75 per cent of the rural people make use of the facilities from the PHCs in Kerala, which is the highest in India (Mahadevan and Sumangala, 1987). As a result of better health care services extensively available throughout Kerala, morbidity, mortality and fertility have rapidly declined. According to the 1981 census, IMR and CBR in Kerala were 37 and 25.6 respectively. Today the crude birth rate of Kerala is equivalent to the level existing in developed countries, but this demographic scenario is not uniform according to the several earlier studies (Kurup & George, 1969; Zachariah, 1983; Kurup,. 1986; Mahadevan, 1986 & 1987) and also the present study. Generally fertility is lowest among the Hindus and significantly higher among the Christians and Muslims. Therefore, the present study considered the major demographic, socio-economic and cultural (Value of children) determinants to explain the existing religious differentials of fertility from a representative region of Kerala, after highlighting their differential social change in Kerala society in general.

2. *Age at Marriage*

Age at marriage forms an important variable that generally regulates fertility. In this context age at marriage of men (27.2) and women (21.9) in Kerala was the highest in India, according to the 1981 census and also during the last four decades. The present data also confirmed the same. The mean age at marriage for women was 19.8 and for men 26.2 years during the time of their marriage, which would have happened at least a decade and beyond. Further, it also varied among the three religious groups; it is somewhat higher among Hindu women (20 years) as against the Christians (18.4 years) and Muslims (17.9). The same trend is also observed for the men. Nevertheless, age at marriage in general showed a negative association with fertility behaviour for the population as a whole and also among the three communities. Therefore, the relatively higher age at marriage of women noticed among the Hindus would have contributed substantially to their lower fertility in contrast to the other two communities.

Certain major determinants of age at marriage have also been studied here; they include: cost of arranging marriage, various reasons for early marriage and late marriage and socio-economic variables. In addition to these factors, occupational mobility and migration also generally contributed to late marriage of girls and boys in Kerala (Zachariah, 1983). Kinship obligation to support the dependent's needs is yet another new and major factor (Mahadevan & Sumangala, 1987). Regarding the cost of marriage, 18 per cent of the population in general spent Rs. 50,000 or more for celebrating the marriage of their daughters. They constitute the highest proportion among the Muslims (44) followed by the Hindus (16%) and a negligible per cent among the Fishermen. While considering various reasons for the determinants of early and late marriage of daughters, significant differences have been observed among the three cultural groups. For early marriage, the Hindus gave less priority. It is evident that education has shown very great influence on late marriage. These determinants are influencing the existing late marriage and low fertility among the Hindus, but not equally so among the non-Hindus. Therefore, suitable steps may have to be taken to increase the age at marriage of Fishermen Christians and Muslims in the light of these findings to reduce their relatively high fertility.

3. *Socio-economic Status Variables*

Socio-economic development of the major communities in Kerala varied not only for the present but also historically. The historical differential opportunities that existed for development among the Hindus, Christians and Muslims during the remote past and particularly the recent past contributed to the different levels of socio-economic development among these groups. From the present empirical findings it was confirmed that the existing differential socio-economic development resulted in differential fertility among these three religious groups. In this context a major social change happened in the family structure. In the past, the joint family was universal, but now the change has been reversed. The present findings also confirmed the same; 61 per cent of the respondents were living in nuclear families as against 17 per cent in transitional and 22 per cent in joint families. Similarly, family structural differences were observed cross-culturally also; while 74 per cent of the Christians were staying in nuclear families as against an almost equal percentage of (57%) Hindus and Muslims. Differences were also observed in their fertility behaviour. It ranges from 2.1 to 3.3 for the joint and nuclear families respectively for the general population. The nuclear families of Christians and Muslims also showed the same rate of fertility; it was however, relatively lower among the Hindus. Thus, the hypothesis confirmed here is that the characteristics of nuclear families contribute to high fertility, irrespective of all the religious groups and especially for the Christians and Muslims. The type of house and electrification of houses showed differences with fertility behaviour for the total population and across these religious groups. Those who were staying in better off (Pucca) houses had the lowest fertility (2.6) as against (3.1) the others, who resided in semi pucca houses. The same trend is observed among the three communities also. Relatively higher percentage of (16.7) the Hindus are staying in better off houses, followed by Muslims (15.9%) and Christians (7.7%). These differences were observed in their fertility behaviour also. But, in the case of electrification, differences in fertility were not significant. Education constitutes the most powerful social variable that explains fertility behaviour all over the world; it has shown, as expected, a negative relationship with fertility behaviour for the total population and for all the three religious groups. Among the three cultural groups, significantly higher proportion of the Hindus have attained higher education, and this leads to relatively low fertility among them. The range of difference in fertility between the illiterates and higher educated women in general varied from 3.9 to 1.2. The corresponding difference in fertility of men's education was from 3.9 to 2.4. From the total findings the hypothesis confirmed here is that education is a major antinatalist factor, which reduces fertility differentially among different religious groups. These findings evidently support the urgent necessity for providing education through different means to these high fertility backward communities like Fishermen and Muslims. Importing formal education requires long term preparation, therefore during a short duration of time, non-formal education may be given the highest priority for the Fishermen and Muslims. Further, the drop out rate of girls from these two communities should also be minimised in schools and colleges.

With regard to occupation, generally women employed outside the home manifest low level of fertility. In the present study, however, an overwhelming percentage of women (76.9%) are engaged in household duties; educated employees constitute only a negligible percentage (3%). Among them Christians and Muslims constitute the lowest number. This is also one of the factors for the low fertility among the Hindus. Regarding occupational mobility, more Muslim men (61.8%) have moved to higher and new occupations, than among the Hindus (48.5%) and Fishermen Christians. It was also noticed that occupational mobility coupled with migration was higher among the Muslims (19%) followed by Hindus and Christians. Here again, those who were employed in Gulf countries manifest the lowest fertility, irrespective of ail the religious groups. Considering the difference in occupational status of wives and husbands together, the hypothesis confirmed is that the couples employed in non-traditional occupations have the lowest fertility, which is true for the husbands employed in Gulf countries, irrespective of the cultural groups.

Economic status historically showed an inverse relationship with fertility, but the present findings did not confirm this trend for the population as a whole fertility is highest among the middle income group (3.1) still less among lowest income group (2.9) and least among the highest income group (2.3). This trend was observed across the three religious groups as well. In this context, among the three religious groups, the largest percentage of Hindus constitute the highest income group, which would have contributed to their lowest fertility. Hence, the hypothesis is only partially proved here.

For measuring the opportunity cost perceived by the respondents, a composite index was developed. On the basis of the index, various costs were classified into three equal groups, which have been designated as low, medium and high categories. From the findings, the level of opportunity cost perceived by the population in general showed a definite negative association with fertility behaviour. It also showed a significant difference in fertility of those who perceived extreme problems of opportunity cost; their fertility ranged from 3.8 to 2.2. The same trend was observed across all the three communities also. Since the Hindus have low fertility, the problem of opportunity cost is relatively less among them. The hypothesis confirmed here is that the increase in perception of different opportunity costs progressively reduced fertility. Taking all the general socio-economic status variables together it is confirmed that couples with better socio-economic status manifest a lower fertility as against their counterparts in the lower strata of society. In this context the Hindus have a better socio-economic status followed by Muslims and Christians. Therefore, their differential socio-economic status also accounts for differential fertility. Urgent attention may have to be given through non-formal education and other economic programmes to improve the social status and level of living of these groups besides modernising them in order to control their fertility.

4. *Value of Children*

Value of children (son) was extensively observed among the total population and the three religious groups. We have identified several dimensions of value of children especially sons. They are economic, social, cultural and psychological values. Among all the nine dimensions of value of children considered here, four of them were found more important for an overwhelming proportion of the total population. These values are: existing children need company (77.9%); economic support during old age (74.6%); salvation of the soul of parents (72.3%) and physical support in the family (71.5%). Among the three religious groups also a similar trend was observed. Out of the extensively confirmed four dimensions of value of children a higher proportion of the Hindus followed by Muslims and Christians manifested these values. According to their order of importance the value of children have increased the level of fertility from 0.4 to 0.7 child when the parents gave importance to these values. Among these three communities also the same trend is observed. For measuring the overall importance of value of son(s) an index was used. All the dimensions of value of children that showed significant influence on fertility behaviour have been used for developing the index. On the whole, according to the degree of importance, the largest proportion of respondents belong to the moderate category (42%). People who attribute high or low values are almost equal (high 30%, low 29%) in their proportions. According to the index, the range in mean live births increases from 2.5 to 3.2, when the importance given to the sons correspondingly increased. A similar trend is observed across the three religious groups also. Those who gave least value show the lowest fertility among the Hindus (2.0) followed by Muslims (2.9) and the Christians (3.1). Hence, the hypothesis is fully confirmed here, that the concept of value of son(s) in general is important for all the population, irrespective of their cultural background, with certain amount of cross-cultural variations on this concept and their fertility. Thus, this factor not only explains the pronatalist influence but also accounts for the differential fertility between the Hindus and non-Hindus.

5. *Breastfeeding*

Breastfeeding is one of the major proximate variables which is universal in this population. Among the population as a whole, an overwhelming proportion (81%) of mother's breastfeed their babies for several months beyond the one month period. While considering the three religious groups, a similar trend is observed. The mean duration of breastfeeding 15.1 months for the total population and 15.7, 15.3 and 14.9 months respectively for the Christians, Muslims and Hindus. In the case of mean duration of amenorrhea period for the population as a whole, it is 7.9 months, and 9.7, 8.5 and 7.9 months respectively for the Christians, Muslims and Hindus. The duration of breastfeeding for the population as a whole and also among the three communities showed a somewhat negative association with fertility behaviour. The difference between the shorter duration of breastfeeding and the longer duration is more conspicuous among the older cohorts in all the communities. It has a greater influence in regulating fertility only among a very small proportion of population, who breastfeed for a very long period in all the three communities. Apparently it does not show much influence in explaining the cross cultural variations in fertility behaviour.

6. *Birth Intervals*

Taking into consideration the closed and open birth intervals together it can be confirmed here that, longer duration of closed birth intervals of three and more years was more among the Muslims followed by the Hindus and the Christians. But on the other hand, the longest duration of open birth interval was more among the Hindus (36.7%) and an equal proportion (27%) among the Christians and Muslims. While closed birth interval influences the formation of low fertility ($\leq$3 children) among quarter of the population also got the benefit of six and more years of duration of open birth interval, which also would have contributed to low fertility for the different cohorts of women. These intervals influenced the differential fertility behaviour of the three communities to a certain extent but not decisively. Because the influence of birth interval might be due to longer duration of breastfeeding and family planning acceptance and not an independent factor by itself.

7. *Contraception*

Kerala is reported to be one of the most successful states in India with respect to family planning practices. About 33.5 (1983) per cent of currently married women have been effectively protected in Kerala as a whole. The present data also confirmed it; an overwhelming (72%) proportion of population of this sample have adopted one or the other permanent or temporary methods of family planning. While considering the situation among the three religious groups, a marked difference is observed across them. The level of adoption of contraception among the Hindus constitutes the highest percentage (78.2%) followed by the Muslims (70.2%) and the Fishermen Christians (57.1%). Therefore, differential adoption of contraception is one of the major factors for the highest fertility noticed among the fishermen and the low level among the Hindus. Among the methods adopted, tubectomy is the most widely used method, irrespective of all the communities and in the total population. An overwhelming percentage (72.2%) of Christians, followed by the Hindus (62%) and Muslims (58%) have adopted tubectomy for the purpose of family planning. It is interesting to note that in case of temporary methods, the Muslims constitute the largest proportion followed by the Hindus and Christians. Regarding the influence of family planning on fertility behaviour there is however, only limited influence. In the population as a whole, those who adopted only the temporary methods alone have slightly less fertility (2.3), but permanent adopters have more fertility (3.4) than even the non-adopters (2.6). The proportion of population who adopted permanent methods out number the temporary and non-adopters of contraception. Therefore, family planning has not regulated fertility at a low level particularly among the overwhelming proportion of permanent adopters. It may be because many of them have taken to sterilization only after reaching the tail end of their reproductive period. Comparing the same phenomenon among the three communities a similar trend is observed except among the older cohorts, of Christians and the younger cohorts of Muslims. Thus, the influence of family planning explains only the limited differential fertility behaviour between the Hindus and non-Hindus.

In addition to the above findings, certain major determinants of family planning have also been identified. Education has shown a direct relationship with contraception at the aggregate level and also across the three religious groups. The findings also proved that the rate of adoption is significantly higher for the low and high parity couple among the Hindus followed by the Muslims and the Christians. Incentives received also showed yet another increase in adoption of family planning. Thus, higher education, incentives and parity constitute the three important factors that regulate family planning acceptance.

8. *Path Analysis*

Thus, out of the six major factors of determinants of fertility behaviour studied here under the path analysis, viz., education, opportunity cost, value of children, age at marriage, breastfeeding and family planning, only the first four factors alone were found to be very crucial in explaining fertility behaviour. These factors also have shown differential influence among the three cultural groups. Education, opportunity cost, value of children and age at marriage, are the most important determinants of fertility behaviour and they also showed differential influence. Therefore, optimum social development coupled with social change particularly on these factors should be emphasized in order to reduce fertility and minimising the cross-cultural variations in natality patterns. Out of the major demographic variables studied, age at marriage emerged as the most important factor followed by family planning. Hence, the new population policy and family planning interventions may have to consider at least these factors to evolve appropriate policies to modify, expand and improve the programme in order to control fertility on a scientific and expeditious basis in this part of our country.

BIBLIOGRAPHY

Agarwala, S.N. 1967: *Effect of a Rise in Female Marriage on Birth Rate in India* : World Population Conference, Belgrade, 1965, Vol. II, New York, United Nations.

Agarwala, S.N. 1964: *Social and Cultural Factors Affecting Fertility in India*, Population Review, 8: 73-78.

Aiya, Nagam, V. 1906: *The Travancore State Manual*, Trivandrum, Travancore Government Press.

Aiyappan, A. 1982: *The Personality of Kerala*, Trivandrum, University of Kerala.

Arnold, F.R.A. Bulatao, C. Buripakdi, B.J. Chung, J.T. Fawcett, T. Jritani, S.J. Lee and T.S. Wu, 1975: *The Value of Children: A cross-national study*. Introduction and comparative Analysis, Vol. I. Honolulu: East-West Population Institute.

Arnold, F. & J.T. Fawcett, 1975, *The Value of Children*, Vol. III, Honolulu, East-West Population Institute.

Audinarayana, N. 1985: *Age at Marriage and its Determinants among the Hindus and the Muslims in Rural Andhra Pradesh*: Ph.D. thesis, S.V. University, Tirupati.

Babbie Earl, 1983: *The Practice of Social Research*, California Wadsworth Publishing Company, Belmont.

Becker Gary, S. 1960: "An Economic Analysis of Fertility". In *Demographic and Economic Change in Developed countries*.

Berelson, B. 1976: The value of children: A Taxonomical Essay in N.B. Tabbot ed., *Raising Children in Modern America Problems and Prospective Solutions*. Bostons, Little Brown, pp. 11-24.

Blake, Judith, 1961: *Family Structure in Jamaica: The Social context of Reproduction*, USA, The Free Press of Glenco, p. 262.

Bongaarts John & R.G. Potter, 1983: *Fertility, Biology and Behaviour: An Analysis of Proximate Determinants*, New York, Academic Press.

Bongaarts, J. 1978: "A framework for Analysing the Proximate Determinants of Fertility", *Population and Development Review*, 41 pp. 105-132.

Bulatao, R.A. & Ronald D. Lee, 1983: *Determinants of Fertility in Developing countries*, Vol. I & II New York, Academic Press.

Bulatao, R.A. 1980: "The transition in the value of children and the Fertility Transition", pp. 95-122 in C. Hohn and R. Mackensen (eds.) *Determinants of Fertility Trends: Theories Re-examined*, Liege, Ordina Edition.

Bulatao, R.A. 1975: *The Value of Children: Philippines*, Vol. II, Honolulu, East-West Population Institute.

Cain, Mead, 1981: "Risk and fertility in India and Bangladesh" *Population and Development review*, Vol. 7 No. 3 New York.

Census of India, 1981: Series - 1, paper 2 of 1983 - *Key Population Statistics Based on 5 per cent sample data*, Registrar General, India.

Chang, C.T. 1979: "Female Employment and Fertility Behaviour", pp. 167-168 in P.J. Chen and J.T. Fawcett, eds., *Public Policy and Population change in Singapore*, New York: Population Council.

Darroch, R.K., P.A. Meyer, & M. Singarimbun, 1981: *Two Age not enough: The value of children to Javanese and Sundanese Parents*, Paper No. 60-D.A., Honolulu, East-West Population Institute.

Davis, Kingslay & Judith Blake, 1968: "Social Structure and Fertility: An analytical Framework" in *Population and Society*, Edt., Charles B. Nam pp. 196-215.

Day, H. Lincoln, 1984: *Analysing Population Trends*, Croom Helm London, Canbera st Martin's Press, New York.

Devan, F. 1977: *Relationship between Advantages and Disadvantages of having children and combinations of desired and actual family size*. Paper presented at the Formal session, Value and cost of children to parents, conference of the International Union for the Scientific Study of Population, Mexico city.

Director of Census Operations, Kerala, Census of India, 1981 Series 10, Kerala, Paper 2 of 1981, Trivandrum, Kerala.

Director of Census of Operation, Kerala, Census of India 1971, Series 4, Kerala & Series-9, Kerala Part II-A, General Pop: Tables, Govt. of India Press.

Driver, E.D. 1963: *Differential Fertility in Central India*, Princeton, Princeton University Press.

Easterlin, R. 1969: Towards a Socio-economic theory of fertility: A Survey of Recent research of Economic factors in American fertility, pp. 127-156 in S.J. Behrman L. Corsa, Jr and R. Freedman eds., *Fertility and Family Planning. A World view*, AnnArbor, Mich. University of Michigan Press.

Fawcett, J.T. 1986: The value and cost of children: converging theory and Research in *Fertility and Mortality*, Eds. by K. Mahadevan, New Delhi, Sage Publications.

Fawcett, J.T. 1983: *Perception of the values of children, Satisfaction and Costs*, Honolulu, East-West centre.

Fawcett, J.T. 1977: The value and cost of children: Converging theory and Research, pp. 91-114 in L.T Ruzicka, Ed., *The Economic and Social Supports for High Fertility*, Canberra, Australian National University.

Fawcett, J.T. (Ed.) 1972: *The Satisfaction and Cost of children Theories concepts, methods*, Honolulu, East-West Population Institute.

Freedman, Ronald, 1986: Theories of Fertility Decline: *In Fertility and Mortality*. (edt.)., by K. Mahadevan, New Delhi, Sage Publications.

Freedman, Ronald, 1975: *The Sociology of Human Fertility: An Annotated Bibliography*, New York, Irwington Publications.

Freedman, Ronald, Parscal K. Whelpton & Arthee Campbell, 1959: *Family Planning, Sterility and Population Growth*, New York, McGraw Hill.

Government of Kerala: *Economic Review, State Planning Board*, Trivandrum (for various years). Statistics for Planning, State Planning Board, Trivandrum (for various years).

Government of India, 1982-83: *Year book*: *Family Planning Programme in India*, New Delhi.

Gulati, Leela, 1976: "Age of Marriage of Women and Population Growth: The Kerala experience", *Economic and Political Weekly*, special number, 11 (31-3).

Gulati, Leela, 1979: "Women and Technological Change. A case study of Three Fishing Villages", *Centre for Development Studies*, Trivandrum.

Iyer, Krishna, L.K.A. 1968: *Social History of Kerala*, Vol. I and II, Book Centre Publications, Madras.

Iyer, Krishna, L.K.A. 1960: *The Cochin Tribes and Castes*, II Vols. Madras, 1901-1912: Travancore, India, *The Travancore State Manual*, 3 Vols. Trivandrum.

Karkal, Malini, 1968: "Age at Marriage", *Journal of Family Welfare*, 14 (3): 51-56.

Kirk, D. 1968: "Factors Affecting Muslem Natality in *Population and Society*, (Ed.) by Charls B. Nam pp. 230-243.

Kiser, C.V. 1960: "Differential Fertility in the United States" National Bureau of Economic Research, Princeton. pp. 77-116.

Kiser, C.V. 1965: "Social, Economic and Religious Factors in the Differential Fertility of low fertility Countries", UNWPC II pp. 219-222.

Koya, S.M. Mohammed, 1983: *Mappilas of Malabar: Studies in Social and Cultural History*, Calicut, Sandhya Publications.

Kurup, R.S. 1986: "Demographic Transition in Kerala" In *Fertility and Mortality*: Theory, Methodology and Empirical Issues edt., K. Mahadevan, New Delhi, Sage Publications.

Kurup, R.S. & George, N.V 1969: "Variations in Fertility between two generations:, *Journal of Family Welfare*, pp. 31-41, 1969.

Kurup, R.S. & George, K.A. 1965: *Population Growth in Kerala Its implications*, Bureau of Economics and Statistics, Trivandrum - 10.

Leibenstein, Harvey, 1974: *The Economic theory of fertility Promising path or Blind Alley*, JEL 12: 457-479.

Leibenstein, Harvey 1957: *Economic Backwardness and Economic Growth*, New York, John Wiley.

Leridon, Hentri, 1977: *Human Fertility. The Basic components*, Chicago, The University of Chicage Press.

Limanonda, Bhassorn, 1983: *Marriage Pattern in Thailand, Rural-Urban Differentials*, Bangkok, Institute of Population Studies, Chulalalongkorn University.

Logan, W. 1987: *Malabar Manual*, Vol. I, Madras, Govt. Press.

Mahadevan, K. & M. Sumangala, 1987: *Social Development cultural Change and Fertility Decline: A Study of Kerala's Fertility change*, New Delhi, Sage Publications.

Mahadevan, K. 1986: *Fertility and Mortality : Theory, methodology and Empirical Issues*, New Delhi, Sage Publications.

Mahadevan, K. 1979: *Sociology of Fertility: Determinants of Fertility Differentials in South India*, New Delhi, Sterling Publications.

Malthus T.R. 1798: *An Essay on Population*, New York, E.P. Dutton.

Mencher, P. Joan & K. Ramanunni, 1975: "Anthropological and Sociological Research in Kerala: Past, present and Future Directions", *In Essays on South India*, New Delhi, Vikas Publishing House.

Mencher, P. Joan 1966: "Namboodiri Brahmins: An Analysis of a Traditional Elite in Kerala", *Journal of Asian and African Studies*, 1: 7-20.

Menon, A. Sreedharan, 1979: *Social and Cultural History of Kerala*, New Delhi, Sterling Publishers.

Menon, A. Sreedharan, 1967: *A Survey of Kerala History*, Madras Vishwanathan (Printers & Publishers) Pvt. Ltd.,

Minkler, M. 1970: Fertility and Female Labour Force Participation in India. A survey of workers in the old Delhi, *Journal of Family Welfare*, 17 (1): 31-43.

Mc Neilly, A.S. 1978: "Effects of Laction on Fertility", *British Medical Bulletin*, 35,2 pp. 151-154.

Nag, Moni, 1972: "Sex, Culture and Human Fertility: India and United States", *Current Anthropology*, 13, 2.

Nag, Moni, 1962: "Factors affecting Human fertility in Non-Industrial Societies: A cross cultural study", Yale University Publication in *Anthropology*, No. 66.

Nair, P.R.G. 1983: "Asian Emigration to the Middle East: Emigration from India, *Working Paper No.180, CDS*, Trivandrum.

Nair, P.R.G. 1981: *Primary Education, Population Growth and Socio-Economic Change*, Allied Publishers.

Nair, P.R.G. 1974: "Decline in Birth Rate in Kerala: A hypothesis about the Interrelationship between demographic variables, Health Services and Education", *Economic and Political Weekly*, 9: 323-326.

Namboodiri, N.K. 1986: "Societal Development and Cultural change: A Reappraisal of selected theories" in *Fertility and Mortality*, edt., by K. Mahadevan, New Delhi, Sage Publications.

Namboodiri, N.K. 1964: "The wives work experience and child spacing, *Milbank memorial fund quarterly*, 42.

Namboodiri, N.K. 1960: *Fertility Differentials and Determinants in Kerala* (Mimeo).

Namboodiripad, E.M.S. 1962: *Kerala, Yesterday, Today and Tomorrow*, Calcutta.

Nayar, P.K.B. 1986: "Factors in Fertility Decline in Kerala" in *Fertility and Mortality: Theory, Methodology and Empirical issues*, edt. by K. Mahadevan, New Delhi, Sage Publications.

Nayar, P.K.B. 1984: "Kerala Women in Historical and contemporary Perspective". *Kerala Women*. Second National conference on Women's studies, Deptt. of Sociology, University of Kerala.

Nayar, P.K.B 1982: *Sociology in India*, Delhi, D.K. Publishing Corporation.

Neuve-La-Louvain, 1983: *Religion and Ideology in Kerala*, Centre de Recherches Socio-Religeus or Universite Catholique de Louvain.

Operations Research Group, 1972: *Family Planning Practices in India*, Baroda.

Population Reports, 1979: "Age at Marriage and Fertility" series No. 4, Baltimore, The John Hopkins University.

Population Reports, 1985: "Mini Laprotomy and Laparoscopy, safe effective and widely used", Baltimore, The John Hopkins University.

Prema, K. & Ravindranath, M. 1982: "The Effects of Breastfeeding supplements on the Return of Fertility". *Studies in Family Planning*, B. 293.

Puthankalam, J. 1977: *Marriage and Family in Kerala*, Alberta (Ph.D thesis).

Paul, Landis, H. & Paul Halt, K. 1954: *Population Problems*, New York, American Book Company.

Rao, M.S.A. 1979: *Social Movements and Social Transformation*, New Delhi, The McMillan Company.

Rao, M.S.A 1957: *Social Change in Malabar*, Bombay. The Popular Book Depot.

Ratcliffe, John, 1978: Social Justice and the Demographic Transition: Lessons from India's Kerala State, *International Journal of Health Service*, 123-144.

Rele, J.R. & Tara Kanitkar, 1980: *Fertility and Family Planning in Greater Bombay*, Bombay Population Prakasam.

Ruth, George, B. Simmons, Gayle, D. Ness & George B. Simmons, 1983: "On the Institutional Analysis of population Programmes", *Population and Development Review*, Vol. 9 No. 3.

Saksena, D.N. 1973: *Differential Urban Fertility*, Demographic Research Centre, Lucknow University.

Schultz, T.W 1973: "The value of children. An Economic Perspective", *Journal of Political Economy* 81 (2 parts).

Srinivasan, K. 1980: "Birth interval Analysis in Fertility Survey *World Fertility Survey Scientific Report* No. 7.

Sinha, J.N. 1967: "Differential Fertility and Family Limitation in an Urban community of Uttar Pradesh", *Population Studies* No. XI, pp. 157-169.

Umadevi, 1984: "Women Education and Employment in Kerala in the Eighties" *Kerala Women*, Department of Sociology, Kerala University.

U.N. 1973: *The Determinants and consequences of population trends*, Vol. I & II New York, pp. 33-63.

U.N. 1975: *Poverty, Unemployment and Development Policy : A case study of selected issues with reference to Kerala*, ST/ESAI, 39, New York.

U.N. 1961: *The Mysore Population Study*, New York.

Vlassoff, M. & Vlassoff, 1980: Old age security and the utility of children in Rural India, *Population Studies*, 34: 487-499.

Whelpton, P.K. & Kiser, C.V. (Eds.) 1946; 1940; 1952; 1954 & 1958: *Social and Psychological Factors affecting Fertility*, Vol. V, New York, Milbank Memorial Fund.

World Fertility Survey 1980: *World Fertility Survey Conference*, Record of Proceeding, Vol. III, London.

World Fertility Survey - Scientific Report No. 71, December 1984.

Wood Cock, George, 1967: *Kerala*: *A Portrait of the Malabar coast*, London, Faber and Faber.

Wyon, B.` & J.E. Gordon, 1971: *The Khanna Study*, Harvard University Press, Cambridge, Massachusetts.

Zachariah, K.C. 1983: *Anomaly of the Fertility Decline in Kerala*, Report No. I, from R.P.O Washington, World Bank.

Index